Integrated Care for the Traumatized

Integrated Care for the Traumatized

A Whole-Person Approach

Ilene A. Serlin, Stanley Krippner,
and Kirwan Rockefeller

ROWMAN & LITTLEFIELD
Lanham • Boulder • New York • London

Published by Rowman & Littlefield
An imprint of The Rowman & Littlefield Publishing Group, Inc.
4501 Forbes Boulevard, Suite 200, Lanham, Maryland 20706
www.rowman.com

6 Tinworth Street, London SE11 5AL

British Library Cataloguing in Publication Information Available

Library of Congress Cataloging-in-Publication Data

Names: Serlin, Ilene A., author. | Krippner, Stanley, 1932– author. | Rockefeller, Kirwan, author.
Title: Integrated care for the traumatized : a whole-person approach / Ilene A. Serlin, Stanley Krippner, Kirwan Rockefeller.
Description: Lanham : Rowman & Littlefield, [2019] | Includes bibliographical references and index.
Identifiers: LCCN 2019013288 (print) | LCCN 2019013553 (ebook) | ISBN 9781538121399 (Electronic) | ISBN 9781538121375 (cloth : alk. paper) | ISBN 9781538121382 (pbk. : alk. paper)
Subjects: LCSH: Psychic trauma—Treatment. | Post-traumatic stress disorder—Treatment.
Classification: LCC RC552.T7 (ebook) | LCC RC552.T7 S47 2019 (print) | DDC 616.85/21—dc23
LC record available at https://lccn.loc.gov/2019013288

Contents

Foreword

That was traumatic! Trauma is everywhere, and the traumatized today are more willing to seek and acquire help compared to a decade ago. Yet, their trauma and its memories are unique to them and must be part of the care they receive. This requires practitioners to view and consider the whole person and their unique experiences and reactions. How one does this is the mission of this book.

I first worked with the traumatized as an assistant professor at Purdue University in 1974. I worked with Vietnam combat veterans who were part of a larger study funded by the National Institutes of Health. I was a researcher, not a counselor. My interest was understanding the trauma induction and reduction process. I did not learn for another eight years while on sabbatical at Princeton that the traumatized had more in common than not, although the causes of their trauma were different. I have also learned that while standards of practice and manualized treatments assure fidelity of treatment, the whole person must be considered for the traumatized, no matter the source of trauma or the treatment of choice.

This is a book about how best to help the traumatized, because the traumatized are those who remain so. Their symptoms include bad memories and other recollections of past events and situations. The traumatized are recovering from an emotional and potentially physical and spiritual shock. Sometimes for the traumatized the shock dislodges their normal and familiar spirituality, their sense of place, their sense of belonging, and, therefore, greater uncertainty. There is considerable pining for their life back and confusion about what has happened to them and why. They want to know how and why they behaved as they did in the thick of the traumatizing event and since then, just as they want to know why they continue to feel obsessed and think about something unceasingly or persistently, and often admit that they "can't get it out of mind." They don't feel safe. Perhaps they feel threatened because they are also thinking, what if the trauma happens again? They have to figure out how best to survive like they did the first time. The traumatized are searching for answers. But they are also searching for security, a sense of safety, for the hope that they can survive and potentially thrive. Thriving is possible with the right help. This book provides a great deal of help for the traumatized.

The author/editors, Drs. Ilene Serlin, Stanley Krippner, and Kirwan Rockefeller, are stellar colleagues, award-winning expert psychologists, and extraordinary and creative trauma practitioners of the whole-person approach. As they note in the first chapter, this approach is a roadmap for practitioners to bring forth, for the clients, as well as practitioners, the best practices not limited to talk therapy. Just as human beings are multifaceted, multidimensional, multilingual, and multiskilled, their treatment should be multimodal, interdisciplinary and multidisciplinary, and flexible so that it fits best with the traumatized and their culture, age, gender, mobility, and preferred mode of communication. As Serlin, Krippner, and Rockefeller point out, a whole-person approach to healing differs significantly from current medical-model practices with the traumatized. The conventional approach focuses exclusively on cause–effect, medicine-focused symptom-reduction. This book represents an alternative to this outdated treatment. The whole-person approach is far more practical. It is grounded in the experiences and preferences of the client.

The whole person includes, of course, everything about them, not just thinking and talking about it. The focus here is on the whole person's mind, body, and spirit. As is noted throughout this book, the whole-person approach to helping the traumatized mediates between cognition and behavior by way of intention, awareness, and mindfulness interventions. Central to this is meaning-making and "existential choice." The traumatized are seeking to get their life back. Their life is more than being obsessed with a traumatizing event and its consequences. But to fully embrace the whole-person approach requires integrated care.

The editors argue that integrated care for the traumatized is the best available approach. Integrated care is like the integrated school: variety leads to better outcomes. Integrated care includes both medical and mental health treatment, prevention programs, and consultation. This kind of care is extremely adaptable to the needs of the client.

The chapters, although written by different experts, sing in harmony to a whole-person approach. The whole-person approach, consistent with integrative care, focuses on designing a treatment plan that addresses the needs of the mind, the spirit, and the body. In chapter 11, for example, Dr. Olweean describes the Catastrophic Trauma Recovery (CTR) Model. It adapts a whole-person approach because it expands the often-narrow perspective of the traumatic experiences of the traumatized. The model protocol guides the traumatized to acknowledge the bigger picture of the traumatizing event, drawing upon the cultural and spiritual elements of the experiences, as well as the cognitive. The model seeks a whole-person perspective as the totality of individuals' traumatic experiences; there is an emphasis on their cultural settings, and the treatment plan includes promoting resilience through building the capacity of their family and community to expand its own self-healing.

Similarly, the whole-person approach is well-illustrated in the chapter by Sword on time-focused therapy. This therapy incorporates critical elements of a whole-person approach in the use of time as a key element of the experience of trauma. Time-focused therapy promotes the healing of survivors through improving insight and skills in self-awareness and self-care. When the time is right, time-focused therapy helps clients reintegrate into society, starting with family and friends.

Another example is the chapter by Dr. Engelman on animal-assisted intervention. It qualifies as a whole-person approach because it enables animals to connect with and calm the client using a biopsychospiritual methodology for reconnecting the survivors with their humanity and restoring their sense of safety and hope.

Science and best practices long ago determined the common and predictable reactions to traumatizing events and traumatic memories. Because we now know what to look for, we can count the trauma in the world and measure its impact on people, families, and communities. Today we know how stress impacts the body, notably the brain, and how best to mitigate the impact. Stress and the psycho–neuro–immunological connections to illness require us to take stress seriously. This is illustrated in several chapters in this book, which have good examples and clinical studies about the role of stress on the brain and body.

Healing trauma comes after facing the unhealed memories in the wake of trauma. Such fields as trauma psychology and traumatology enable us to understand the risk and protective factors in managing traumatic stress reactions. This book applies the emerging knowledge to help practitioners help the traumatized.

This book will promote healing in the traumatized by educating practitioners in alternative approaches to those found today because a better approach to helping the traumatized requires it. The whole-person approach within an integrative care context is an important innovation that should be taught to anyone who works with, or may work with, the traumatized, starting with reading this book.

Charles R. Figley, PhD
Kurzweg Chair in Disaster Mental Health and Distinguished Professor
Tulane University Traumatology Institute
Tulane University School of Social Work

I

Foundations

Chapter One

The Whole-Person Approach to Integrated Health Care

Ilene Serlin, Stanley Krippner, and Kirwan Rockefeller

A whole-person approach integrates the best of psychological practices into an integrative biological/psychological/spiritual/social model, which encourages prevention, resilience, and self-care. This approach, which relies on experiential, as well as theoretical, learning, uses symbolic and nonverbal, as well as linear and verbal, modes of thought and expression (Frewen, Brown, & Lanius, 2016). A whole-person approach to healing represents a paradigm shift from an illness, symptom-reduction, medical model to a growth, meaning-enhancing, integrative model. This approach incorporates intention, awareness, and mindfulness as the mediating variables between cognition and behavior. It includes the areas of meaning, beliefs, and existential choice. From this confrontation with mortality can come a renewed will to live (Serlin, 2007).

When people are faced with issues of trauma and consideration of life and death, the topic of spirituality inevitably comes up. Understanding that people are cultural and spiritual beings is a necessary condition for a psychology of human existence (Sue, Bingham, Porche-Burke, & Vasquez, 1999, p. 1065). A whole-person approach honors the spiritual dimension of life.

Trauma is often preverbal and nonverbal, carried through nightmares or the body's reactions. It includes such somatic and mind–body symptoms as headaches, physical pain, numbness, withdrawal, hyperarousal, digestive problems, and fatigue. Expressive arts, symbolic movement, and mindfulness meditation help to express the story that is carried in the body; they can also help contain and transmute the participant's experience through verbal and nonverbal narratives. With the courage to create (May, 1975), new narratives can evoke a self that moves from deconstruction to reconstruction (Feinstein & Krippner, 1988; Gergen, 1991; May, 1989; Sarbin, 1986).

As we, the editors, experienced work throughout the world from holistic perspectives, we wanted to share this work, showing that working models have been established, writing about the research that has been done, and advocating for more exploration and research. These methods have been shown to be powerful, but they need further development and training. We hope that this book will stimulate interest in following them up with further studies.

The first question usually raised is that of evidence, as in: Show us the evidence that whole-person approaches work. The second chapter, therefore, confronts the question of evidence in the evaluation of whole-person models, in acknowledgment of the need to have valid outcome assessments. Focusing on the case for methodological diversity in the study of trauma treatments, the chapter offers a critique that "trauma" and resilience are often studied as decontextualized variables, rather than as lived phenomena to be investigated with regard to the existential meanings they hold for individuals. As the medical and psychological communities have recognized the need to provide more person-centered care, research methods specifically capable of holistically investigating the lived experiences of military trauma and resilience are required. This may be particularly true in the military setting, where soldiers are sensitive about receiving mental health diagnoses (Meredith et al., 2011) and at risk for misunderstanding and stigma.

This chapter provides an overview of the phenomenological method, an approach to qualitative research that has been developed to allow for contextualized knowledge of personal life experiences and faithfully honors and offers understanding of the individuals who are being studied (Wertz, 2015). In this chapter, the philosophical and historical roots of phenomenology are outlined, followed by a description of the method itself and how it has been applied in social science research based on the extensive work of Giorgi (2009). Examples from the authors' study of military resilience in Israel animates the discussion of this methodology, its applicable procedures, and its illustrative findings when used to explore the lived experiences of military servicemen.

A working model of a whole-person approach can be found in chapter 3, which outlines a seven-step Integrative Healing Model, a holistic approach to healing trauma with a mind–body–ecospirit emphasis. Meaningfulworld's humanitarian outreach programs focus on national and international trauma, violence, and mediation through missions conducted in more than 45 nations and 30 states in North America. At the core of the programs is the seven-step Biopsychosocial and Ecospiritual Model, through which various aspects of trauma, disputes, conflicts, disagreements, or the impact of disasters are assessed, identified, explored, processed, worked through, and released. This process transforms trauma and suffering by offering new meanings or new lessons learned. This innovative model incorporates various theories. These include the psychodynamic (Freud, 1910); the interpersonal (Sullivan, 1953); the existential and humanistic (Frankl, 1962); electromagnetic field balancing (EMF, Phoenix Dubro & Lapierre, 2002); forgiveness and reconciliation (Kalayjian & Paloutzian, 2010); learning theory, flower essences, essential oils, and physical release (Van der Kolk, 1987); mind–body–spirit chakra balancing; prayers; and meditation. The outcomes of the use of the seven-step Integrative Healing Model have been measurable, and survivors have reported experiences of being empowered, healed, strengthened, at peace, and able to overcome their negative reactions to the trauma. They have also related having embraced healthy coping patterns, which improve their ability to prepare by staying centered and empowered with new and positive lessons learned. Beginning with interpersonal healing, the seven-step Integrative Healing Model addresses the transformation and collaboration so profoundly needed by our world as it moves through violent transitions; moreover, the model demonstrates the interconnectedness of our interpersonal healing and development, conflict transformation, happiness and well-being, and inclusive and sustainable community building.

Another area of study in terms of whole-person approaches to trauma is the highly important work with children. Research shows that children suffer considerably postdisaster, both immediately and in the long term. Chapter 4 describes a model of psychosocial support for children that integrates simple techniques leading to resilience and empowerment through the creative arts. The model addresses key constructs in disaster recovery, including safety and strength-building, as well as songs, drawings, and constructions, including objects circulated among various cohorts in different countries. The model has been applied in numerous settings and cultures, including postearthquake in Haiti, after the tsunami/earthquake in Japan, and during the Ebola epidemic in West Africa. Key lessons learned are described. Trainings were given to local volunteers to conduct the sessions for the children and provide sustainability of the service. Cultural adaptations were made for each situation. Despite the limitations of conducting research in disaster conditions, data supporting the impact of the training in some settings are included.

Some successful programs of working with refugees and trauma are based in the arts. In a program carried out in Istanbul and Bangladesh, dance movement therapy (DMT) was a primary component of the healing arts program. Chapter 5 explores how DMT, as part of an integrated treatment model used in Istanbul to work with Syrian refugees, can be a powerful tool for social change. DMT as a creative arts therapy complements traditional verbal psychotherapy to build healthy connections on both personal and social levels, using the body as a container for the emotions and memories of individuals who have experienced traumatizing events or posttraumatic stress disorder (PTSD). The ability to make healthy decisions and develop resilience in the midst of difficult life circumstances is a central theme of this work, as these people generally have difficulty establishing their personal boundaries, trust, and communication. As violence is often reciprocated throughout the lives of children and adults who have experienced traumatizing events, DMT offers a safe way to respond to these intense emotions, allowing for their expression through nonviolent means. According to a wide range of research, DMT helps to enhance a wholesome approach to the integration of body and mind within both individuals and the social environments they create. By establishing a sense of safe space using ground rules and a predictable structure, DMT can go beyond the limits of verbal language and its barriers by creating a new group language that is nonviolent and expressive. Emphasizing the power of choice and control over participants' responses to their interactions with family, friends, and other members of the community, DMT seeks new ways for building peace and understanding in times of chaos.

While most whole-person models involve human beings, some of them are discovering that nonhumans may be able to address the preverbal and shattered communicative challenges faced by the traumatized. Chapter 6, on animal-assisted interventions (AAI), explores various animal-assisted programs currently in practice, as well as the theory and research related to the psychophysiological benefits of AAI. One startling number indicates that 7.8% of the U.S. population is affected by PTSD; however, averaging the percentages of PTSD found among veterans from the Vietnam, Gulf, Afghanistan, and Iraqi wars indicates an even higher percentage of 18.3%. Given that such conventional treatment methods as exposure and cognitive-behavioral therapy are not always effective, the focus of this chapter is on an alternative and integrative model of PTSD treatment using AAI.

The chapter begins with a discussion of PTSD, including the DSM-5 defining criteria, rates of occurrence of PTSD derived from military service, and problems with traditional treatment methods. Then the treatment alternative of AAI is introduced. This includes its definition; the history of its use in treating PTSD (plus the Veterans Administration's restriction on its use); the different roles animals may play in helping those with PTSD; and, most important, the proposed mind/body/brain mechanisms of action underlying AAI's successful use in helping PTSD sufferers. The chapter presents an innovative theoretical model explaining AAI's success in the treatment of veterans with PTSD, who may experience a multitude of problems, including dissociation, social isolation, numbing, nightmares, intrusive thoughts, suicide, and vast physical health problems, together with pain. To help "reset" the nervous system by means of a more holistic approach, it is proposed that AAI makes use of specific integrative healing dimensions operating through the mind/body/brain connection. These healing factors psychophysiologically soothe people with PTSD and help them return to feeling safe in their bodies and their lives. The specific healing elements and concepts in AAI that are elucidated include prosodic modulation, neuroception, vagal toning, hypnoanalgesia, neurofeedback, and biofeedback (heart rate variability and physiological entrainment). The paradigm that incorporates these theories and mechanisms of action draws upon previous models espoused by well-known researchers Drs. Stephen Porges (polyvagal theory) and Bessel van der Kolk, among others. One case vignette is included to demonstrate how these psychophysiological concepts are implemented in clinical practice.

Another arts-based approach to working with the traumatized is one based in the dramatic arts of storytelling, or drama therapy. The Therapeutic Spiral Model (TSM) is a clinical system of experiential change that integrates classical psychodrama, gestalt therapy, and playback theater. Drawing on recent research on the effects of war at different levels of human functioning, from neurobiology and attachment theory to paradigm shifts in social and political movements, TSM has been for many decades a leader in the field of alternative therapies for people with PTSD. The neurobiology of trauma shows that new learnings can actually change the brain following experiences of war, as well as other traumatic events in individual, family, and societal life. What the action methods of change have in common is that they rely on the creation of spontaneous new experiences as the curative agent of change, making it a perfect match for effective and targeted treatment of the impact of war on the lives of people throughout the world.

Chapter 7 also presents an overview of the basics of classical psychodrama, gestalt therapy, and playback theater as long-used alternative methods of change. While TSM has been used for therapeutic, as well as structural, change, it is always clinically based on attachment theory, using the Trauma Survivor's Intrapsychic Role Atom (TSIRA) to guide the necessary safety and containment to prevent retraumatization for people affected by war and its multidimensional impacts. The TSIRA provides a map delineating the roles internalized by trauma and those needed for healing. Research on TSM with female Iraq War veterans previously diagnosed with PTSD are presented, showing improvements in self-esteem, family connections, and empowerment. Additionally, the use of TSM to prevent secondary PTSD in the Third Division of the Chinese Army, first responders to the 2008 earthquake in Chengdu, China, are presented. Examples of the use of TSM with refugees in the sociopolitical conflict between Palestine and Israel, as well as a program for sustainability training for refugee counselors in Egypt, are also documented.

Many approaches to therapy and self-help focus on people's history, emphasizing how past events adversely affect their thought processes. Unfortunately, reliving past traumas or unhappy experiences can have extremely negative effects. For instance, one may be stuck between a traumatic "past negative" experience and one's hopeless "present fatalism." If such individuals do think about the future, it is usually in negative terms. In time perspective therapy (TPT), discussed in chapter 8, the focus is on balancing people's past negatives with positive memories of the past and their present fatalism with some present hedonistic enjoyment; then plans are made for a bright, positive future. TPT is another holistic, goal-oriented talk therapy, a fast, easy, and effective approach that works both in clinical settings and as a self-help tool. It helps individuals gain internal balance, as well as balance in significant relationships, socially, and in the work place. TPT switches the focus from past to present, from negative to positive, clearing the pathway for the best yet to come: the future. TPT has proven effective for a wide range of people, from seasoned war veterans and survivors of accidents, assault, abuse, and neglect, to individuals, couples, and families searching for a new way to handle the ever-increasing stress of day-to-day life and problematic situations. When our time perspectives—how we view the past, present, and future—are skewed, usually in the negative, not only are we affected, but also the people with whom we come in contact: family, friends, and coworkers. TPT helps people see patterns they may have adopted as coping mechanisms for living with stress, anxiety, depression, day-to-day struggles, and worries. It shows them how to help themselves, as well as their loved ones.

Trauma psychology in the United States has been critiqued for focusing on the individual, whereas other countries, especially non-Western ones, understand trauma more in terms of communities. What is the damage to the community, and how can it be healed? Chapter 9 presents a model of community work to prevent and treat trauma in Israel. The state of Israel, which was established in 1948, after the Holocaust, was immediately forced into a war of independence (leading to a loss of 1% of the population). Since then, Israel, which has continued to exist under constant threats, has been forced to cope with recurrent wars and ongoing terror attacks. In this ongoing traumatic reality, and under the shadow of a massive collective trauma, NATAL (Israel Trauma Center for Victims of Terror and War) was established in 1998. It is an apolitical nongovernmental organization (NGO) that aims to serve as a multidisciplinary therapeutic home for trauma casualties related to the Israeli–Arab conflict. NATAL is directed by a comprehensive professional philosophy, addressing the various circles of traumatic impact on individual casualties and their families through a unique help line, along with traditional clinical staff; it also involves the wider community through an outreach unit operating to prevent and reduce traumatic impact, promote resilience, and conduct emergency interventions. In addition, NATAL incorporates mental health professionals through its trauma-focused psychotherapy school and Israeli society at large through a public relations and communications unit operating to increase visibility, awareness, and legitimacy of the discourse regarding war and terror-related trauma.

Throughout the years, more than 200,000 Israelis have been helped by NATAL. In this chapter, the professional activities and operating philosophy of the various units are described and demonstrated through case studies, showing the best practices and interunit cooperation leading to optimization of treatment. Within this framework, the main elements of NATAL's unique model are discussed, namely: a multiprofessional, humanistic, and holistic approach; emphasis on continuity of care; and addressing various target populations from the individual casualties and their relatives, through the community under threat, to the society as a whole. The authors also address the traumatic timeline: promoting resilience and raising preparedness ahead of time; encouraging real-time interventions; and treating posttraumatic casualties. A central aspect of NATAL's view and model is to address trauma through two prisms: the personal, individual trauma, alongside the trauma of the collective ("national trauma"). In this context, the authors offer the possibility of considering trauma as a potentially uniting bridge, which can promote understanding, acceptance, and opportunities for the two societies, Israeli and Palestinian, which are wrapped in the chains of their mutual trauma, while yearning for a peaceful resolution.

Community-based healing rituals are found not only abroad, but also in the United States, with indigenous healing psychotherapy and restorative circles. Western psychotherapy's mainstream approaches to treating trauma focus primarily on individuals' problems and pathologies, which often means ignoring the larger interpersonal and historical contexts that contribute to human thought and action, including the transmission—and healing—of trauma. Katz (2017) refers to the healing wisdom of indigenous people as the "first psychology." In his view, indigenous psychology focuses on issues of community building, interpersonal relations, and spiritual understanding. Most indigenous psychotherapies close the gap between individual and larger community contexts by viewing trauma in more holistic terms, seeing it as the loss of one's soul, along with the disconnection of relationships among self, others, and the larger circle of life. Indigenous people, in general, view the effects of trauma on an individual as being communal and spiritual, as well as personal. Chapter 10 is an exploration of how these concepts have resulted in communal healing when applied in culturally relevant ways to address trauma resulting from youth and gang violence.

Community-based healing practices also address cultural belief systems and their impact on trauma. These belief systems, which help us make sense of our everyday experience, can also help us make sense of trauma. Approaches to healing acute trauma require an appreciation for the multifaceted and multidimensional experiences of our individual reality, our sense of self, our identity, and, by extension, the realized experience of our relationship to the world and our place in it. The field of philosophy has held a continual dialogue on this most unique quality and characteristic of being human—our unavoidable preoccupation with being engaged daily in making sense of our reality, of creating meaning in our lives. In chapter 11, from the time of our earliest ability to detect and absorb sensations as human beings, we are busily engaged in collecting, analyzing, and forming meaning about what is happening in and around us. As these meanings about life events interact with our most fundamental needs, the reactions amalgamate into beliefs about our reality, throughout time codifying into belief systems that set the frame of reference for the world in general. The positive to negative qualitative nature of those beliefs defines the context of what we can expect of ourselves, others, and the world. Since profound trauma permeates every dimension of an individual's reality, along the way previously secure positive beliefs can be severely shaken, or even shattered, to be replaced by debilitating and damaging negative beliefs and fragmented perceptions of reality that color the experience of day-to-day life from that point onward.

On the communal level, the process is vastly more complex, as legacies of unresolved communal trauma become embedded in the group ethos and are passed on to future generations as transgenerational trauma to serve as fuel for polarization, war, and violence, both within and between communities. Healing entire communities requires innovative adaptations and scaling up of whole-person approaches. This chapter examines the unique multidimensional dynamics and challenges of individual and communal trauma, offering Common Bond Institute's integrated catastrophic trauma recovery (CTR) model as an example of a successful whole-person approach to trauma-informed treatment in promoting healing, reintegration, resilience, and growth at both the individual and communal levels.

What is the future of integrative care? One new area of discovery is that of caregiver burnout and compassion fatigue. Since Charles Figley has opened the door to an exploration of burnout and secondary trauma, chapter 12 continues the examination of caregiver satisfaction and regeneration. A multimodal model for promoting these goals is presented, drawing upon the perspectives of attachment theory and the "broaden and build" theory of positive emotions, as well as on research on compassion fatigue and satisfaction. This approach, developed in SELAH, the Israel Crisis Management Center, aims to enhance a sense of hopefulness, connectedness, and meaning through tapping into helpers' strengths, rather than focusing exclusively on stress management or symptom relief. Initially developed to support a network of 600 volunteers providing emergency support in the aftermath of terrorist attacks and other crisis situations, this model has been applied by different trauma organizations in Israel. It uses outdoor and nature-based experiential activities with mindfulness training, narrative practices, and verbal and nonverbal creative modalities, creating a wide spectrum of opportunities for self-expression, cultivating compassion for self, and sharing. Caregiver burnout and compassion fatigue are receiving significant attention from health professionals, but the current literature has focused almost exclusively on the negative consequences of caregiving at the expense of exploring the entire spectrum of the caregiving experience. This chapter focuses on pathways both of preventing burnout and compassion fatigue and of promoting caregiver satisfaction and regeneration. Since the multifaceted nature of the caregiver experience calls for an integrative perspective, the whole-person approach is a particularly relevant framework due to its integration of cutting-edge practices into a bio/psych/spiritual model supporting prevention, resilience, and growth. It represents a paradigm shift away from an illness orientation to a growth-oriented model. The struggle with adversity may lead to the discovery of strengths and enhancement of life's meaning. Witnessing human suffering can take a toll on one's resources, but it can also lead to a renewed sense of purpose.

Had we more space and time, we could have collected many more whole-person approaches to integrative health care; however, the chapters in this book make the case that holistic treatment is already functioning quite well in a number of settings. We hope they will inspire practitioners to treat survivors of trauma holistically, as whole people, and not as mere statistics or labels. The number of traumatized people grows daily. Their future—indeed the future of the world—depends on how they can be guided toward recovery, resilience, and growth.

REFERENCES

Feinstein, D., & Krippner, S. (1988). *Personal mythology*. Los Angeles, CA: Jeremy P. Tarcher.

Frankl, V. (1946/1962). *Man's search for meaning*. Boston: Beacon.

Freud, S. (1910). The origin and development of psychoanalysis. *American Journal of Psychology*, *21*(2), 181–218.

Frewen, P. A., Brown, M., & Lanius, R. (2016, May). Trauma-related altered states of consciousness (TRASC) in an online community sample: Further support for the 4-D model of trauma-related dissociation. *Psychology of Consciousness: Theory, Research, and Practice*, *4*(1). doi: 10.1026/cns0000091.

Gergen, K. (1991). *The saturated self*. New York: Basic Books.

Giorgi, A. (2009). *The descriptive phenomenological method in psychology: A modified Husserlian approach*. Pittsburgh, PA: Duquesne University Press.

Kalayjian, A., & Paloutzian, R. (2010). *Forgiveness and reconciliation: Psychological pathways to conflict transformation and peace building*. New York: Springer.

Katz, R. (2017). *Indigenous healing psychology: Honoring the wisdom of the first peoples*. Rochester, VT: Healing Arts Press.

May, R. (1975). *The courage to create*. New York: Bantam.

May, R. (1989). *The art of counseling*. New York: Gardner.

Meredith, R. W., Janečka, J. E., Gatesy, J., Ryder, O. A., & Murphy, W. J. (2011, October). Impacts of the cretaceous terrestrial revolution and KPG extinction on mammal diversification. *Science*, *334*(6055), 521–24.

Phoenix Dubro, P., & Lapierre, D. P. (2002). *Elegant empowerment: Evolution of consciousness*. Ashland, OH: Platinum Publishing House.

Porges, S. W. (2011). *The polyvagal theory: Neurophysiological foundations of emotions, attachment, communication, self-regulation*. New York: W. W. Norton.

Sarbin, T. (ed.). (1986). *Narrative psychology: The storied nature of human conduct*. New York: Praeger.

Serlin, I. A. (2007). *Whole-person healthcare: Vol. 3: The arts and health*. Westport, CT: Praeger.

Sue, D. W., Bingham, R. P., Porche-Burke, L., & Vasquez, M. (1999). The diversification of psychology: A multicultural revolution. *American Psychologist*, *54*(12), 1061–69.

Sullivan, H. S. (1953). The interpersonal theory of psychiatry. New York: W. W. Norton.

Van der Kolk, B. A. (1987). The drug treatment of posttraumatic stress disorder. *Journal of Affective Disorders*, *13*(2), 203–13.

Wertz, F. J. (2015). Phenomenology: Methods, historical development, and applications in psychology. In J. Martin, J. Sugarman, & K. Slaney (eds.), *The Wiley handbook of theoretical and philosophical psychology* (pp. 85–101). Hoboken, NJ: Wiley.

Chapter Two

Methodological Diversity in the Study of Trauma Treatments

Batya Rotter and Frederick J. Wertz

As a whole-person approach to treating individuals who have experienced difficult life events, this chapter focuses on the questions of assessment and empirically based understandings of "trauma" and "resilience" as constructs used in research, as well as diagnoses to inform clinical treatment planning. In the research world, studies of trauma and resilience often fail to convey the complexity or nonverbal nature of trauma, as well as the processes that shape its unfolding and resolution. The reason is quite clear: "Trauma" and "resilience" are studied as decontextualized variables that hold no meaning within the life-world of participants. We offer a case for methodological diversity in the study of "trauma" and "resilience," and show how these constructs can be investigated as lived phenomena, including the existential meanings they hold for individuals. As the research world informs clinical practice, offering an evidence base to guide clinical judgment and develop clinical interventions, we suggest that a more holistic practice for studying and measuring trauma-related constructs is necessary to understand the experiences and human responses that are targeted in treatment of the whole person.

What is the experience of trauma and resilience like? How is it lived and experienced? The phenomenological method is an approach to qualitative research that has been developed specifically to allow for contextualized knowledge of personal life experiences; it faithfully honors and offers a generalized understanding of the individuals who are being studied (Wertz, 2015). In this chapter, we briefly discuss the philosophical roots of phenomenology and explore the method itself, based on the outline by Giorgi (2009). Examples from our study of military trauma and resilience in Israel will animate the discussion of this methodology and its applicable procedures, and how it allows for an understanding of the lived experience using the whole-person approach.

ASSESSMENT AND METHOD: WHY THEY MATTER

Symptom checklists and diagnostic criteria allow researchers and clinicians to identify elements of a phenomenon uniformly. Yet, if understanding is not founded on actual human experiences, one can miss how these symptoms are meaningfully organized in the context of psychological life. This is especially true in an era when empiricism has become a hypothesis-testing procedure, and randomized controlled studies have turned into a process in which isolated variables are correlated to predetermined outcomes without positing a meaningful interrelationship between them. A brief look at the scientific literature on military resilience can help illuminate how the whole-person approach, through a focus on lived experiences, can widen the empirical landscape to deepen understandings of trauma and resilience-related phenomenon.

One problem with the randomized-control literature on military resilience is that resilience has often been operationalized and measured by what it is not—the absence of clinical trauma symptomatology. This binary approach to measuring resilience stands against findings that veterans endorse both positive and negative appraisals of combat experiences, suggesting that well-being may be marked by the simultaneous presence of both positive and negative sequelae; moreover, it may additionally be thought of as existing on a continuum (Aldwin, Levenson, & Spiro, 1994; Elder & Clipp, 1989; Southwick et al., 2014). In addition, by studying military resilience using hypothesis-testing methods, researchers have been forced to define and measure trauma-related constructs in narrow ways that may be far removed from the contextually meaningful experiences of individuals. Many studies of trauma and resilience, for example, focus on the abstract relationship between predictors and outcomes, without addressing the fundamental psychological questions of why these relationships exist and what meaning they hold for the individual. This point was raised in an open conversation at the 2018 American Psychological Association conference, where prominent trauma researchers discussed how the new DSM-5 diagnostic criteria for PTSD do not speak to the severity, duration, or intensity of the traumatizing events, nor the meanings these life events hold for various populations (Resick et al., 2018). Such discourse begs the question of how the human experience sheds light on phenomena as they are lived and what methods, aside from hypothesis testing, are available to assess this meaning and inform clinical practice.

An additional critique of hypothesis-testing research methods is found in postmodern and poststructural theories, which posit that knowledge is created through discursive language that must include the voices of research participants. Conversely, the absence of participants' voices essentially denies them the right to coconstruct knowledge about their own well-being, which may actually harm the participants in the long run (Martineau, 1999; Ungar, 2004). Similarly, it has been argued that definitions of *resilient behavior* are too focused on a Western definition of *health*, and that cultural and contextual factors play an important role in how well-being after trauma is experienced (Ungar, 2008). Such arguments suggest that, if we continue to focus on posttrauma symptoms without understanding the contextual, cultural, and psychological significance they hold for individuals, we may not only misdiagnose them, but also not fully understand and thereby disempower those who we seek to support.

PHENOMENOLOGY AND THE WHOLE PERSON APPROACH

Phenomenological research methods provide the tools to describe the experience of a psychological phenomenon without preconceived scientific and positivistic suppositions, making it a methodology that is uniquely suited for exploring the emergent constituents and structure of combat trauma and resilience in natural settings. In addition, the practice of phenomenology demands that the researcher be immersed within the world of the person/participant to understand the phenomenon in question. In this manner, it offers a unique way to explore whole-person meanings and experiences of combat trauma and resilience. In phenomenological research, results are described in a way that make sense according to the research questions and subsequent data, often in the present tense (as a phenomenon that is still occurring).

In our study with 14 Israeli (male) combat veterans aged 23 to 45 years, we described our findings using a temporal structure, mapping the developmental progression in which young Israeli men engage during the different stages of service: preconscription, basic training, combat, discharge from the military, and homecoming/civilian integration. We chose a temporal sequence, because we found that understanding the experience of resilience and trauma at each developmental juncture required an appreciation of the experiences that preceded it. For example, we described the naïve position of the preconscript, one who has not yet engaged in combat but is motivated by the meanings of service he has received from his social context (brothers, fathers, neighbors), meanings that speak directly to his yearning to make something of himself (e.g., establish his place within his family, community, and nation). Describing the position of the preconscript is important, because it contextualizes the motivation and guiding social messages that he brings into military life, and sheds light on the progression that shapes his ability to withstand the challenges of both military life (where he must give up his individuality and independence) and the life-threatening conditions of combat (where he may give up his life).

As another example, we noticed that to understand how a young civilian becomes a soldier ready for combat, we needed to understand that he undergoes a spatial, temporal, and relational repositioning during basic training and acculturation to military life. Here his spatial life shifts from civilian living to the military base, and his temporal awareness shifts to "military time." As his life becomes more conscribed within the physical and temporal world of his military existence, so, too, his relationships are shaped by the ideals and priorities of military goals and his allegiance to his comrades. Only by distancing himself from his preconscription/civilian identity and position can he intuit that the collective is more important than the individual (the military ethos of "we-ness"), as well as develop an orientation of ever-readiness, an allegiance to his military cohort (*Hev'reh*), and a trust in his military superiors—constituents that are imperative for his successful fulfillment of military missions and even survival in combat. Thus, in the context of understanding what trauma and resilience mean to a soldier, we first had to enter his world and see it through the temporal, developmental, spatial, relational, and embodied layers that comprise his psychological life. By entering into his world, we adopt a whole-person lens to see the many facets of his lived psychological experience, from which we glean insights and descriptive clarity about the phenomenon in question.

Case examples from phenomenological research are important to understanding how the method is applied in practice (see Wertz et al., 2011). In the next sections, we consider some phenomenological procedures and illustrate them through case examples from our study with Israeli combat veterans. Our goal here is not to map *all* the developmental processes, but rather to highlight a *few* processes, with a focus on the phenomenological method. In addition, while our study encompassed the many different phases of military service, due to the scope of this paper we have limited our examples to the basic training and combat phases of military life. (For an exposition of post-combat experiences of homecoming resilience and trauma, see Rotter, 2015.)

Beginning the Practice of Phenomenology: Intentional Analysis of Meaning Units

Attentiveness to psychological meanings and the ability to conceptualize their essence is not uncommon in everyday life. Indeed, these processes are employed by many psychologists informally and as part of their training; however, these processes are made explicit and rendered as the focus of a research method by phenomenologists, and the procedures have been codified as a scientific method that can be taught, trained, practiced, and improved with education and mentorship. There are resources to guide the novice practitioner that outline step-by-step approaches, the most notable of which is Giorgi's *The Descriptive Phenomenological Method in Psychology* (2009), where he outlines a method for the empirical (data-based) study of psychological phenomena. As one might expect from a whole-person research method, the way in which research is conducted must honor the participants and remain faithful to their voices. Raw data are collected in the form of descriptions or interviews in which open-ended questions lead to various concrete descriptions of lived experiences that are then analyzed.

A sound phenomenological study starts with collecting detailed data that are concrete and revelatory of lived experience. In our study, we interviewed 14 combat veterans, asking them to narrate their experience of transitioning from military to civilian life, from the beginning to the end, describing concrete examples of real-time events where they experienced well-being or distress. During these semistructured interviews, we encouraged participants to provide a comprehensive narrative without commentary or general musings (based on theories, diagnosis, or research) to describe situations, feelings, relationships, and experiences as they were actually lived (see Rotter, 2015). Sometimes we asked for more description ("Tell me more about that"), so as to elicit additional descriptive data that would allow us to enter into their life-world and experience their narrative alongside them.

In the first step of analysis, to apprehend the holistic meaning of the participants' descriptions, we read (and reread) the interview transcripts and occasionally relistened to the audio recording of the interview to recall the nonverbal expressions (e.g., pauses in narrative, laughter) in the interview. One hallmark of this open-reading stage of analysis is the attitude of *psychological phenomenological reduction*, where the researcher approaches the subject matter with an open attitude, seeing the examples with fresh and naive eyes to explore the meanings of situations as experienced by the research participants (Wertz, 2005). In addition, through reading, we began to couple open attentiveness with a psychological focus, in which we reflected on the described experience with a focus on the very meanings experienced by the participants as they lived them—in this case, experiences of resilience and trauma; technically, this is the beginning of a process called *intentional analysis*, an explication of meaning, about which we speak more throughout the chapter.

When reading the transcripts, we began to take note of moments within the text that contained psychologically meaningful descriptions that were constitutive of, or relevant to, the lived experience of trauma and resilience. These segments of description are called *meaning units*; once they were identified, we reflected on how they provided important insights into the participant's world of trauma and resilience (Giorgi, 2009). The following is an example of a meaning unit from the beginning of an interview conducted with Eric, a combat soldier who engaged in three high-artillery/deadly encounters and experienced clinical symptoms of both trauma and recovery:

> I was actually at a Hebrew Language Immersion program, and a representative of the army came to speak to all the men. All the students were saying, "So what is the army going to do for me, how much is the army going to pay me, what am I going to get out of doing it?' I was just really embarrassed. There were a lot of terror attacks going on then, and I just said, "Where can I sign up, how quickly can I sign up?" . . . I was embarrassed by their lack of sense of responsibility, their sense of entitlement to be rescued from their financial situation without having to secure a home for ourselves. . . . Yeah, I felt like I had to at least pull my weight; if I have to stand on somebody else's shoulders, then I need to let somebody else stand on mine, too.

Here Eric expresses his goal structure and values, namely, that he is strongly committed to contributing to the well-being of the collective he is joining and takes great pride in the purity of his dedication to the great cause of a homeland, of which he intends to be a part, as something very good, something to which it is worth devoting his life. At the same time, there is an awareness of alternative reactions, ones that seem to Eric selfish or noncollective, and here we can see Eric's idealism of right and wrong, good and bad.

A number of procedures are used in the reflective explication of meaning units enacted in *intentional analysis*, which are described in detail by Wertz (2011). They include 1) empathetic immersion in the descriptions; 2) slowing down to dwell on experiential moments described in the text; 3) magnifying and amplifying what was described; 4) becoming intensely interested in the experiences being described; and 5) focusing on the significance (or meanings) of experiences, rather than the experiences themselves. In addition, the researcher must keep in mind the research topic, so that meanings and reflection direct focus toward the phenomenon in question. For example, Eric's sentiments appeared to be relevant to his experience of trauma and resilience, as they included the ethos of the preconscript, someone who is an outsider to the military system, not yet a soldier and not yet living in the confines of a military base. This outsider-ness brings with it a position of unknowingness that defines the preconscript's idealistic framing of military life. This position is contrasted by the moment he enters the military:

> The day I went into the army, draft day, I don't know how much they meant for it to be this way, but it was a pretty shocking experience. You really become a number; whether they meant to do this or not, they communicated pretty clearly that now I am the property of the army. I understand that not everybody has to do this, but I had to write letters to people that they would get

> if I'm killed and things like that. It's not like it's fun, but I figured I was pretty prepared for that.

There is a psychological shift that took place on conscription day, when Eric became a number and spatially relocated from the world of civilian living to the military base. He reported the experience of joining the collective (an ideal in his preconscription phase) as a shocking act of disautonomy, one in which he loses ownership of his selfhood. Even his life is something he must write away in a letter, giving it to his military superiors to hold for him; symbolically, this is giving over control, as well as entrusting the military body to protect his life and those of the men around him, while they in turn protect the nation.

We reflected on this meaning shift and the significance it held for Eric on his continued journey through the military, and what these experiences indicate about his encounter with trauma and resilience. We noted that he must let go of some civilian sense of independence and change his own relationship with the military; on the one hand, he was shocked that he had to write a letter in the event of his death, but in the next breath he had to fully accept and prepare himself for it ("I guess I was pretty prepared for that."). This is a moment of acculturation and submission, a complete modal shift into soldierness, for which there is no space or time for dissonance, hesitation, or regret. Indeed, as we reflected on the many instances Eric described about entering military life and the subsequent experiences when he feels resilient or vulnerable, we identified a common demand to shift adeptly away, to disconnect, from civilian life and to achieve a sense of congruence with a newly emerging soldier mode of life.

FROM INDIVIDUAL TO GENERAL ANALYSIS: AN EXAMPLE OF SOLDIER MODE

Reflecting on meaning-units allows the researcher to create individual narrative summaries based on each participant's descriptions and analyses. Here, *intentional analysis* is enacted to deepen individual descriptions with psychological insights that hold meanings about the phenomena of trauma and resilience. Once this individual level of findings is completed for several participants, the researcher can begin general analyses in which the various narratives are compared, with a distinct effort to understand what is essential, or invariant, to the structure of the phenomenon in question across multiple examples. This process, which is called *eidetic analysis*, informs us of the generality of essential moments and their meanings at various levels. At the idiosyncratic level, the researcher describes what is invariant among the multiple experiences of each participant, the constituents and organization of each individual's unique trauma and resilience. At the typical level, the researcher describes constituents and structures that occur in a subgroup, although not involving all participants (from which one can identify "types"). Finally, at the highest level of generality—that which is experienced by all participants—the researcher delineates the invariant constituents and structure of all examples of the phenomenon. It should be noted that, at each level, the researcher considers empirical variations from collected data, as well as imagined and otherwise known variations, to grasp the essences of individual, typical, and highly general experiences.

The process of generalization requires that the researchers compare narratives, identify essential themes, and reflect on the structural organization of the constituent themes. One highly general and essential constituent of military resilience and trauma that we found was the embodied position of what we have called *soldier mode*, which we conceptualized through multiple narratives that described this position and its importance for psychological life in combat. For example, Marc described the way he seamlessly shifted into a combat position and assumed a machine-like stance to enter the combat zone:

> And then our officer comes and says, "Two minutes, everyone get into gear." And at that point you don't think, you are like a machine. The head officer came and spoke to us, and we were doing our routine and prepping. They gave us very little information. They told us that another unit was stuck and we needed to go in and help them. And then we started moving.

His machine-like quality allowed him to be a vehicle without a civilian conscience, to enact orders without thinking, and to focus on mission success by way of routine. We see how his combat goals were manifested in both gear and action, serving as a holistic unity, in that his gear offered him the physical protection and method of attack for the sake of accomplishing his unit's collective combat goals. This stance was further evidenced when a grenade fell right in front of him, failing to explode on impact, during his first moments in combat:

> Grenades were falling all around us, and I remember one landed right in front of me, but it didn't explode. I looked, and I was like . . . um . . . but you don't have time to think. You just go, you are like a machine, you just continue. . . . That's something I remember very clearly—the first day, the walking. We walked for 14 hours into the combat zone.

Here, he was so completely focused on his mission that he did not commemorate or contemplate the miraculous moment when his life was spared. Instead, he continued walking with resoluteness; his machine-like quality precluded experiencing any fear of his mortal vulnerability as he moved forward with an unflinching, robotic, and unstoppable presence. Because the combatant has practiced being in an embodied soldier position during military training, soldier mode in a combat mission has already become a familiar, routinized way of being.

For example, when Sam witnessed the carnage caused by a mortar landing during his first moments in combat, he entered a novel scenario, but his training dictated his actions such that he never lost his combat position:

> I didn't drop anything, I just ran forward, with all my things still on me. I ran forward and started patching them up, the way you have been taught to. You take out your bandages or anything you've got on you . . . and you do that with every single one of them, you keep running back under fire, until you get all of them out.

The immediacy of his response belies the experience of familiarity with his soldier calling, as well as his ability to completely embody the intention of his service: protection of others-as-his-nation. He acted as a matter of routine, pulling out bandages and running back and forth with wounded soldiers on his back. Soldier mode afforded him the visceral bodily action stance with an attitude of at-homeness within the combat setting, without thinking, just doing what he was "taught to do."

What makes soldier mode an essential constituent of military resilience? Throughout our reflections, we used *free imaginative variations*, where the researcher imaginatively plays with different descriptive conceptualizations that capture the essential invariant psychological features and organization of the data, until a structure that best fits the data is developed. For example, we imagined that combat would be existentially terrifying for a civilian, but, in contrast, soldiers who had developed a soldier mode described combat as a challenge ripe with opportunities for transcendent meaning and goal fulfillment. A person in soldier mode welcomes the opportunity to initiate and actualize military goals in every empirical and imaginable combat situation. For example, when Dean learned that his unit, stationed at the border of a combat zone, would not enter to fight, he expressed a feeling of dismay, a "moment of anticlimax." Similarly, Zack described that he was upset when he sustained an injury, because "I was itching to go into combat. I wanted to do what I was there to do. I mean, you are trained to do something—you want to use it." Any imaginable soldier familiar and comfortable with this position yearns to actualize what he is capable of doing, and this sense of mastery and capability is what allows him to enter combat and face any conceivable threat, hardship, injury, and pain with resilience. Indeed, soldiers look forward to engaging in combat missions as a way to break up the monotony of military life, which has its reason for being and fulfills its most important goals only in combat.

Ami, for example, described the heighted visceral feeling of attunement he experienced in combat as compared to other duties on the base, describing combat as arousing and enlivening. He shows that an important element of combat resilience entails the ability to not only make a home and familiarize oneself with the embodied combat stance, but also embrace and enjoy this milieu as "home." This constituent of resilience is evidenced by the decision some soldiers make to extend their military service beyond their mandatory call to duty, where, despite exposing themselves to more combat risks, they find enjoyment, meaning, or satisfaction in their military activities related to the fact that they now *belonged* in combat ("I knew my trade, and I was a good soldier"). These feelings of familiarity and mastery that are experienced in the combat "home" are essential to military resilience, because they foster congruence between a soldier's being and his military goals/actions, a complete alignment between a soldier mode of being and the combat situations he faces.

Exiting Soldier Mode: Understanding Combat Vulnerability and Wounds

If soldier mode is considered a protective position of psychological survival, due to the sense of combat embodiment and familiarity that it affords the soldier who must complete his mission, then the movement of *exiting* soldier mode deprives the soldier of this comforting protection, leaving him vulnerable, exposed, incongruous with his context. Here we continued to use intentional analysis (How does this description relate to distress in combat?) and eidetic analysis (How does this description express and illuminate something highly general, typical, or idiographic about distressing moments in combat?) to describe moments in combat that are revelatory of trauma and resilience.

The following are examples from Eric's combat tour, as well as other soldiers' experiences, which show how moments of *exiting* during service lead to profound and poignant moments of *combat vulnerability*, when the soldier engages in thoughts or reflections that concern his existential being on a civilian level. These examples of combat vulnerability reveal nonresilient moments insofar as the soldier leaves soldier mode and experiences some form of mental or physical paralysis that hinders his ability to complete his combat tasks with embodiment and familiarity.[1]

After his unit was attacked during routine guard duty, Eric was injured, and his close friend was killed. While in the hospital recuperating, he *exited* soldier mode, instead experiencing vulnerability, self-doubt, concerns about his actions vis-à-vis his comrade, and concerns about his comrade's family. The first manifestation of *exiting* appears in his description of silence in the hospital, a dramatic depotentiation of action, wherein he is literally unable to utter a word to a single person: "I wasn't able to talk for a couple of days—

not that I couldn't speak about what happened, I just couldn't speak at all." Here, removed from a combat context, he is no longer in his combat stance, that automatic, familiar, navigable engagement toward the goal of a military mission. His encounter with his comrade's deceased parents at a memorial ceremony presented another *exit*, as he moved out of the immediate and present-focused orientation of combat and focuses on the past, where he experienced anxiety and engaged in prolonged reflections about combat (including self-doubt) outside a combat setting:

> We went to visit my friend's parents. My friend being killed was more traumatic [than my injury]. . . . What was hard was facing his parents. I know that in the end of the day they wouldn't have really blamed me, but they still might have blamed me, they still might have looked at me in their pain and said, "Why couldn't you have moved him over a bit more?" or whatever. And in my own little analysis, by the way, he was in a place behind me, where he was actually more safe than I was, and so when I pulled him down with me under the truck to protect him, I actually made him unsafe. But, I mean, what can you do?

Here, he straddled the military and civilian worlds—he was a soldier, but he exited soldier mode and was now engaged in civilian interactions that left him raw and vulnerable, paralyzed and speechless. How could he explain to civilian parents what happened in combat? After this encounter, we see him feeling dangerously incongruent with his soldier persona, where he engaged in a ruminative focus on himself in an effort to examine and find justification for his past combat actions. His silence can thus be understood as an act of distancing himself from others, because he deemed himself unfit to speak or interact with other humans while he contemplated how he might have killed a fellow comrade, essentially failing to be a "good soldier."

It is important to note that *exiting* movements threaten a soldier's efficacy and ability to complete his combat assignment with automaticity, precision, familiarity, and embodiment. We see this in another life-threatening mission, when Eric *exited* soldier mode again and experiences a form of paralysis that placed both himself and his comrades in danger:

> And my friend is slapping me in the face. I was, like, "What?" I was a little confused, and we'd been getting shot at for a couple of minutes, and I kind of blacked out, I was terrified, I was just . . . my friend slapping me in the face telling me that we need to come up with a plan, we need to do something. . . . I don't think I fainted; I just looked into space and went somewhere else in my head, I guess. That was really scary. . . . The fact that these young men are going to sit there paralyzed until I'm commanding them, that they are not going to do anything until I'm awake—that was really scary, pretty horrifying.

In this episode, Eric *exited* his soldier position while facing a combat situation and became incapacitated, requiring a member of his unit to slap him in the face to rouse him from a paralysis. This is another situation in which he failed to protect, thereby actually endangering his comrades, which to him was "pretty horrifying."

We found that moments of *exiting* soldier mode left soldiers with a sense of vulnerability that made it difficult to move back into a combat position; often they were remembered as *combat wounds*. Daniel exemplifies both these features, where he had difficulty repositioning back to soldier mode after he left combat to attend a fallen comrade's memorial service. First, he described feelings of vulnerable incongruity, which constitutes an *exit* when witnessing soldiers in uniform express civilian emotions: "To see men crying, as opposed to seeing soldiers gnarling—it was strange." This "strangeness" is on account of seeing soldiers, who are meant to embody a military ethos and abstain from civilian emotion, engage in precisely those civilian emotions of pain, grief, and existential insecurity. Second, once he exited, he expressed the difficulty he had returning to his military position: "[Back at the base], we had a very, very, very hard time. We all just felt empty and spent. Like when we saw the graves, it was very hard to go back." Here, he struggled to deal with civilian emotions while still carrying the responsibility of being a "good soldier"; as a result, he was unable to reconcile the incongruity of the two worlds he was straddling, making it difficult to shift between the two. Third, the memories from his *exit*, far from leaving him, in fact, cause him continued emotional distress in the form of a traumatic dream during the night he spent at his parents' home after the funeral: "I woke up in the middle of the night from a dream where people were insanely shooting at me, and I fell off the bed." Thus, one can see how the prolonged duration of his encounter with the civilian world when *exited* from soldier mode created a psychic space in which he experienced emotional vulnerability and pain in both dream life and waking life. In this way, *exiting* soldier mode allows for experiences of emotional upheaval that threaten a soldier's resilience during his service, even as it threatens his ability to remain focused on combat tasks and shift back into a position of soldier mode embodiment. Furthermore, *exiting* soldier mode had implications for Daniel's postcombat adaptation to civilian life, as the vulnerabilities he experienced in a military and combat setting changed the course of his resilience narrative once he became a veteran (see Rotter, 2015).

It should be noted that soldiers recognize the dangers of *exiting* soldier mode in combat contexts and work hard to avoid exiting hazards. For example, many soldiers mentioned that they had the option to call their family members while stationed in enemy territory, but they chose not to do so, because their overwhelming desire to adopt the role of a son (a civilian role) would inhibit their ability to act as a machine in combat. Michael described a visit from his parents on the base as follows: "It was nice to see them, but it was also not so nice. It left me with a bad feeling, because, in order to be in a good position for fighting, you have to be disconnected from what you are leaving behind at home. It made it harder for me to cope." These soldiers show how even small opportunities to *exit* soldier mode were perceived as dangerous, because they threatened to remove the soldier from his alignment with his combat mission and compromised his ability to return to a sense of oneness with his military life.

DESCRIBING AND UNDERSTANDING RATHER THAN DIAGNOSING AND INTERVENING

Clinicians have always known that ailing people are experiencing more than just symptoms. For a scientific community striving for practices that speak from a whole-person perspective, it is clear that other kinds of evidence must become part of the empirical lexicon. This is especially true in the field of psychology, where concrete, personal psychological life experiences should be the focus of empirical understanding and addressed in treatment. Phenomenological structural knowledge is descriptive, differing from a clinical diagnosis or dictionary definition in that it is long, in-depth, and multidimensional, aimed at fostering understanding of the many constituents and layers of lived experience. Using a phenomenological method with all its descriptive richness and analytic tools (e.g., open reading, identifying and reflecting on meaning units by means of intentional analysis, comparing real and imaginal variations of narratives using eidetic analysis) allowed us to map how soldiers are a distinctive population in the way they live through trauma and resilience, because they are active agents who undertake risk as a project that is supported by social values and has meaning within their military and national contexts. Sharing examples from the combat phase of our study, we explored how soldier mode develops as a soldier's preconscription ideals and motivations shift into a military phase, during which time a soldier learns to develop a mode of being designed to help him remain focused on military goals, psychologically shielded from concerns and matters of civilian life.

In the combat context, we described how soldiers could act as "good soldiers" to achieve resilience by adopting and embodying soldier mode, where they can do what they are trained to do with mastery and feelings of congruence or at-homeness. By contrast, soldiers described moments of suffering and distress in combat as experiences of *exiting* soldier mode, where they were unable to animate their military mission due to feelings of disconnect, incongruence, paralysis, and confusion.

We thus found that an essential constituent of the phenomenon of combat resilience in relation to trauma is the ability to shift, adapt, or move flexibly between soldier and civilian modes of being. A related constituent is the ability to recognize when such shifting, or difficulty in shifting, serves important and meaningful functions in the person's life as a whole—the life in which one is both soldier and civilian.

There are many facets of our study that we are unable to share here due to the constraints of space, as well as the more paramount interest in describing the phenomenological method. Here we hope to convey how, to meaningfully understand the experience of resilience and trauma for combat soldiers and veterans, one must map the whole person's lived experience and understand the temporal and developmental progression of that experience. To do this we open ourselves up to the experience with fresh eyes; push our comprehension to understand narrative with a psychological focus; and compare narratives with an eye to discerning what is highly general, typical, or unique about this experience in relation to a larger phenomenon.

Husserl described the "ego-act-object" structure of consciousness, in which he argued that there can be no meaningful definition of a phenomenon without describing its essence as a psychological experience by returning to the individuals who live through the intentional mental activity. Phenomenologists do this by returning to the narratives of the individuals who experience the phenomenon firsthand in their multifaceted and complex psychological lives, and by using analytic techniques that describe the temporal, developmental, spatial, relational, and embodied dimensions of psychological life. The whole-person approach requires that we focus on what Husserl called the "life-world"—the world of lived experience that precedes research and contains an inexhaustible richness of human meaning, in contrast to a reduction of the person's engagement in the world to symptoms or diagnoses that hold no contextual meaning in real life.

REFERENCES

Aldwin, C., Levenson, M., & Spiro, A. (1994). Vulnerability and resilience to combat exposure: Can stress have lifelong effects? *Psychology and Aging*, *9*, 34–44.

Elder, G. H., & Clipp, E. (1989). Combat experience and emotional health: Impairment and resilience in later life. *Journal of Personality*, *57*(2), 311–41.

Gade, D. M. (2013, Summer). A better way to help veterans. *National Affairs*, *16*. Retrieved from http://www.nationalaffairs.com/publications/detail/a-better-way-to-help-veterans.

Giorgi, A. (2009). *The descriptive phenomenological method in psychology*. Pittsburgh, PA: Duquesne University Press.

Martineau, S. (1999). *Rewriting resilience: A critical discourse analysis of childhood resilience and the politics of teaching resilience to "kids at risk."* Unpublished doctoral dissertation. Vancouver, Canada: University of British Columbia.

Resick, P., Fairbank, J. A., Schnurr, P. P., & Keane, T. M. (2018, August). Evolution of PTSD as a diagnosis: Perspectives from experts in the field. In D. T. Castillo (ed.), *Conversation hour, trauma psychology, division 56*. Conducted at the American Psychological Association (APA) Annual Convention, San Francisco, CA.

Rotter, B. (2015). *Resilience of Israeli soldiers in transition from military to civilian life: A phenomenological study*. Doctoral dissertation. ProQuest Dissertations Publishing, 3728446.

Southwick, S. M., Bonanno, G. A., Masten, A. S., Panter-Brick, C., & Yehuda, R. (2014). Resilience definitions, theory, and challenges: Interdisciplinary perspectives. *European Journal of Psychotraumatology*, *5*(1), 1–14.

Ungar, M. (2004). A constructivist discourse on resilience: Multiple contexts, multiple realities among at-risk children and youth. *Youth & Society*, *35*(3), 341–65.

Ungar, M. (2008). Resilience across cultures. *British Journal of Social Work*, *38*, 218–35.

Wertz, F. J. (2005). Phenomenological research methods for counseling psychology. *Journal of Counseling Psychology*, *52*(2), 167–77.

Wertz, F. J. (2015). Phenomenology: Methods, historical development, and applications in psychology. In J. Martin, J. Sugarman, & K. Slaney (eds.), *The Wiley handbook of theoretical and philosophical psychology* (pp. 85–101). Hoboken, NJ: Wiley.

Wertz, F. J., Charmaz, K., McMullen, L., Josselson, R., Anderson, R., & McSpadden, E. (2011). *Five ways of doing qualitative analysis: Phenomenological psychology, grounded theory, discourse analysis, narrative research, and intuitive inquiry*. New York: Guilford Press.

NOTE

1. When these moments of vulnerability persist in his civilian life through vulnerable combat memories, he is considered to have *combat wounds*, which are the emotional vestiges of pain and incapacities accrued in combat that are incongruous with the person's goals as he turns to engage in civilian life. Combat wounds are alluded to in this section, but they could not be fully discussed due to space constraints (see Rotter, 2015).

II

Whole-Person Group Therapy Models

Chapter Three

The Seven-Step Integrative Healing Model

Ani Kalayjian and Daria Diakonova-Curtis

MEANINGFULWORLD

The idea of treating the whole person is gaining momentum among healing professionals. Although these specialists are still generally trained in one area only, there is a growing shift in the field to viewing healing as multidisciplinary and holistic, involving many aspects of the human experience. This chapter describes the work of one organization, the Association of Trauma Outreach and Prevention (ATOP), termed *Meaningfulworld.* Its approach to healing trauma applies a mind–body–ecospirit method, through which various aspects of trauma or conflict, or the impact of disasters, are assessed, worked through, and released. This process transforms trauma and suffering by offering new meanings or new lessons.

Founded in 1990 and affiliated with the United Nations, ATOP Meaningfulworld has committed itself to the service of humanity by creating healing, instilling peace, and transforming generational pain and suffering. The organization uses state-of-the-art scientific theory, as well as peace and consciousness research, to promote the education and skill development of mental health professionals, teachers, arts therapists, alternative medicine practitioners, clergy, nurses, mediators, and laypersons working in communities affected by trauma. Meaningfulworld's Humanitarian Outreach Programs have been established in more than 45 countries throughout the world in seven regions—Africa, Asia, North and South America, the Caribbean, Europe, and the Middle East—transforming the lives of more than 1 million people. For two and a half decades, Meaningfulworld has been on a journey of healing that has focused intensely on how forgiveness and meaning impact levels of trauma and resilience. Much of this work has taken members of Meaningfulworld to places where healing has been the focus of professional and scientific work, engaging many people in these countries.

Meaningfulworld's mission is to help develop a meaningful, peaceful, and just world where everyone can enjoy good mind–body–ecospirit health. Meaning is nurtured through a process of learning, reflection, and mindfulness that transforms old habits through new experiences with a sense of responsibility. This is facilitated by healthy relationships that foster honest and open communication, with love and spiritual connection, working toward an ultimate goal of a peaceful and meaningful global society (www.Meaningfulworld.com).

Monthly workshops in New York City, in addition to humanitarian outreach programs abroad, are some of the ways Meaningfulworld accomplishes its goals. Workshops are offered to community members, professionals, and paraprofessionals. Humanitarian outreach programs are carefully organized according to a systematic approach in response to such current traumatic events as a natural disaster or human-made crises. For example, members of Meaningfulworld were on the ground in Puerto Rico only weeks after Hurricane Maria devastated the island in 2017. Other humanitarian missions were conducted following an earthquake in Haiti, a civil war in Burundi, and political unrest in the Middle East. Working with individuals who have lived through devastating events like hurricanes, earthquakes, and even war requires a whole-person approach, because it is necessary to address the mental, physical, and spiritual effects of such trauma on the individual, the community, and the Earth.

At the heart of Meaningfulworld's work is the seven-step Integrative Healing Model, through which traumatic experiences are assessed, explored, released, and eventually reintegrated. The model builds upon the integration of multiple theories, including the following: psychodynamic (Freud, 1910); interpersonal (Sullivan, 1953); existential and humanistic (Frankl, 1962); forgiveness and reconciliation (Kalayjian & Paloutzian, 2010); learning theory, flower essences, essential oils, and physical release (Van der Kolk & Saporta, 1993); and soul-surfing (Kalayjian, 2015), prayers, and meditation. The seven steps of the model include 1) assessing levels of distress, disagreement, or conflict; 2) encouraging the expression of feelings; 3) providing empathy and validation; 4) encouraging discovery and expression of meaning; 5) providing information; 6) instilling eco-centered healing; and 7) learning breathing, movement-centered healing, and meditation. This model provides the basis for the humanitarian outreach missions of Meaningfulworld (Kalayjian, 2002; Kalayjian & Sofletea, 2012).

At the core of the healing practices is Meaningfulworld's view that recovery following trauma is achieved primarily through two psychological processes: meaning-making and forgiveness. The ability to find meaning in the traumatic event and cultivate a sense of purpose in life has been described as one of the central components of healing from disasters (Frankl, 1962; Kalayjian & Eugene, 2010a, 2010b). Meaning-making has been linked to better adjustment following stressful life events (Collie & Long, 2005; Skaggs & Baron, 2006) and lower severity of posttraumatic symptoms (Kalayjian, Shigemoto, & Patel, 2010).

The catalyst of Meaningfulworld's model is forgiveness (Frankl, 1962; Toussaint, Kalayjian, & Diakonova-Curtis, 2017). Forgiveness provides the necessary cognitive, emotional, and spiritual space and resources, as well as the appropriate shift to present and future perspectives, to bring about meaning in life and reduce trauma symptoms (Frankl, 1962; Toussaint, Kalayjian, & Diakonova-Curtis, 2017). Forgiveness can alleviate suffering by changing the past, not as a record of actual events that occurred, but through reappraising its meaning in the present (Roxberg et al., 2010) and cocreating a healthy future. Both forgiveness and meaning-making improve not only mental well-being, but also physical health and spiritual connectedness.

The following section provides a detailed account of how the seven-step Integrative Healing Model is applied during Meaningfulworld's healing workshops. One or two leaders follow the seven steps below, while guiding the group through the steps.

THE INTEGRATIVE HEALING MODEL

Step 1: Assessing Levels of Posttraumatic Stress

The first step requires an assessment of the group and its level of distress following a devastating event. Participants are given the Harvard Trauma Questionnaire (HTQ) to determine severity of trauma, followed by questionnaires on forgiveness and meaning-making to assess how these practices have impacted the levels of trauma. The HTQ, which assesses both perceptions of actual trauma events (including torture) and symptoms associated with trauma, has been translated into many different languages. Its psychometric properties have been deemed reliable across different cultures. There are 16 questions related to the participants' experiences and symptoms of trauma, for example, "Do you feel depressed?" "Do you have nightmares?" and "Are you worried or nervous?" The participants respond to the statements on a Likert scale ranging from 1 (not distressed at all by the symptoms) to 4 (extremely distressed) (Kleijn, Hovens, & Rodenburg, 2001).

The Meaning in Life Questionnaire, which is used to measure the search for meaning and the presence of meaning in one's life, consists of 10 questions, with the responses based on a seven-point Likert scale (Steger et al., 2006). Participants indicate how true the statement is for them, from 1 (absolutely untrue) to 7 (absolutely true). An example of a question related to the *search* for meaning in life is, "I am seeking a purpose or mission for my life," while an example of a question related to the *presence* of meaning in life is, "I have a good sense of what makes my life meaningful." Forgiveness is measured by the forgiveness subscale of the Brief Multidimensional Measure of Religion and Spirituality, which contains single items related to forgiveness of self, forgiveness of others, and feeling forgiven by God. The three items are as follows: "I have forgiven myself for things that I have done wrong," "I have forgiven those who hurt me," and "I know that God forgives me" (Fetzer Institute and National Institute on Aging Working Group, 1999). Responses are collected anonymously and with informed consent. The questionnaires are used to collect data about a group for the purposes of understanding the current group dynamics and overall level of trauma to tailor the healing workshops to the needs of that particular group and its members.

Step 2: Encouraging the Expression of Feelings

The group leader then encourages one or multiple participants (one at a time) to express their feelings in the "here and now," as related to the disaster they have experienced. Release of feelings is therapeutic, as it helps lessen the grip the trauma has on us, enabling us to let it go. Participants are encouraged to follow the model known as IDEAL: Identifying the emotions; Describing the feelings connected to the event, rather than the event itself; Expressing the feelings (becoming familiar with naming the particular emotions, as well as identifying physical sensations related to the feelings); And, finally, Letting go.

Step 3: Providing Empathy and Validation

The workshop leader then encourages group members to provide validation to the person who shared in step 2. Survivors' feelings can be validated by the members using such statements as "I can understand . . ." or "It makes sense to me . . . ," and sharing information about how other survivors from throughout the world have coped. It is important to provide members with a sense of support and encouragement for meaning-making during a difficult time. Also used is *intentional therapeutic touch*, for instance, holding a survivor's hand. Here it is reinforced that the survivor's feelings of grief, fear, and frustration about the situation may turn into anger, if not processed. Group members are provided with an "Anger Wheel" of emotions to help them make connections between anger and other underlying emotions, for example, sorrow, anxiety, or disappointment. We also encourage expression of positive feelings of joy of survival. When this model is practiced individually (not in a group setting), people are encouraged to find an empathic and nonjudgmental person with whom to share their trauma and from whom to accept empathy.

Step 4: Encouraging the Discovery and Expression of Meaning

During this phase, group members who have shared are asked, "What lessons, meaning, or positive associations did you discover as a result of this disaster?" This question is based on Viktor Frankl's logotherapeutic principle that a positive meaning can be discovered in the worst catastrophe. Group members are encouraged to share lessons learned and any meaningful connections achieved during the previous steps. Focusing on positive outcomes, personal strengths, and new possibilities is known to increase posttraumatic growth and resilience by decreasing such negative emotional responses as hopelessness, anger, and distress, according to research cited by the American Psychological Association (Collier, 2016).

Step 5: Providing and Gathering Information

Next, practical tools and information are given on how to overcome the effects of trauma, including the use of a systematic desensitization process. The importance of preparation for natural disasters and mindfulness regarding human-made traumas is reinforced. Disaster preparedness is discussed and elaborated. Information regarding forgiveness and self-healing is shared, including relevant books, articles, movies, and any useful materials. Group members are encouraged to share with one another tools and resources that have helped them in the past.

Step 6: Using Eco-Centered Processing

In the last two steps of the Integrative Healing Model, participants are encouraged to think beyond themselves to increase their sense of connectedness with humanity, the Earth, and, if appropriate, a spiritual sense of the universe. Practical tools are shared to connect with Mother Earth. Discussions and exercises are conducted around environmental connections. Ways to care for one's environment are shared, starting with one's personal surroundings and expanding to the larger globe, learning about how we can impact our environment and how the environment, in turn, impacts us. Here, awareness of Mother Earth is presented as a way to heal oneself and others. Connecting with the sunrise and sunset, identifying with trees and flowers, and merging ourselves in the ocean or sea can cleanse both our bodies and our souls.

Step 7: Finishing with Breath Work, Movement Exercises, and Meditation

Finally, breath is used as a natural medicine and a healing tool. Since trauma can confront individuals with a loss of control, survivors are assisted in discovering ways of controlling their own responses. They learn how to use breath for self-empowerment, moving thereby to release fear, uncertainty, and resentments. In addition, they use exercises to practice gratitude, compassion, and forgiveness in response to disasters. Breath work is combined with a series of physical movements that mindfully focus on each energy center, its color vibration, its use, and its benefit, balancing and energizing each center with affirmations specifically designed for it. This combination of movement, color identification, evaluation of the physical area, affirmation, and breath is called *soul-surfing.* The Integrative Healing groups conclude with a Heart-to-Heart Circle of Gratitude and Love, in which participants join hands in a circle and place their joined hands over the heart of the person to the right. This provides attendees with the opportunity to experience a sense of connectedness with one another, people throughout the world, and all humanity.

Overall, the workshops provide participants with a whole-person approach to healing from traumatic events, as different aspects of the human experience, including emotions, physical sensations, meaning-making and lessons learned, and eco and spiritual interconnectedness are touched upon and reinforced. These techniques particularly address the whole person by allowing participants a safe space wherein to focus on various aspects of their individual posttraumatic experiences. Participants are taught how to pay attention to not only their thoughts and emotions, but also their body sensations, breathing, and relationships with others, as well as look beyond themselves to the earth and to the universe. The outcome is measurable, as participants have reported experiences of being empowered, healed, strengthened, at peace, and able to overcome their negative reactions to the trauma (Toussaint et al., 2017). They have also reported having embraced healthy coping patterns, which in turn have improved their ability to prepare for future adverse events by staying centered and empowered on the basis of new and positive lessons learned.

Beginning with interpersonal healing, the Integrative Healing Model addresses the transformation and collaboration so profoundly needed by our world as it continues to move through violent transitions. Moreover, it demonstrates the interconnectedness of our interpersonal healing and development, conflict transformation, happiness and well-being, and inclusive and sustainable community building. Each of the seven steps follows evidence-based theories, for example, encouraging the expression of feelings (Freud, 1910), providing empathy and validation (Sullivan, 1953), encouraging discovery and expression of meaning (Frankl, 1962), facilitating forgiveness and reconciliation (Kalayjian & Paloutzian, 2010), instilling eco-centered healing, and demonstrating breathing as a form of movement-centered release (Van der Kolk, 1987).

Any adult with a desire to offer healing in a postdisaster area can be trained to become a workshop facilitator. ATOP Meaningfulworld offers such a certification program consisting of eight daylong training events in New York City, concluding with a graduation ceremony at the United Nations. More information about the training program can be found at http://meaningfulworld.com/our-work/workshops.

Meaningfulworld has worked in more than 45 countries and more than 25 states in the United States, paying close attention to the cultural needs of each country or state. The workshop materials have been translated into several languages, including Spanish, Armenian, and French Creole, and it has employed translators and cultural insiders to give participants the chance to express their thoughts and emotions in their native language. Furthermore, due to the organization's commitment to social justice and partnership with the United Nations, workshops have been conducted to illuminate gender-based variables that contribute to horizontal manifestation of trauma, for instance, domestic violence. Finally, to ensure that this work is sustainable and lasting, Meaningfulworld outreach teams continue communication with the collaborations and connections made during trips and workshops. Post-workshop follow-up with facilitators and, in some cases, the participants is an essential step in ensuring that the changes are lasting. Meaningfulworld teams have also organized follow-up trips to such countries as Puerto Rico, Haiti, and Armenia to reevaluate and reassess the needs of the community following the original program. Data are collected at follow-up and, when appropriate, compared with the original data. Generally, a decline in post-traumatic symptoms and an increase in meaning-making and forgiveness are observed throughout time.

CONCLUSION

Complex trauma that addresses multicultural and multigenerational issues needs a whole-person approach. Meaningfulworld builds on an integration of established and alternative methods to address the bio–social–spiritual and ecological needs of traumatized people throughout the world.

REFERENCES

Collie, K., & Long, B. C. (2005). Considering "meaning" in the context of breast cancer. *Journal of Health Psychology*, *10*, 843–53.

Collier, L. (2016). Growth after trauma: Why are some people more resilient than others—and can it be taught? *American Psychological Association Monitor on Psychology*, *47*(10), 48.
Fetzer Institute and National Institute on Aging Working Group. (1999). *Multidimensional measure of religiousness/spirituality for use in health research*. Kalamazoo, MI: Fetzer Institute.
Frankl, V. (1946/1962). *Man's search for meaning*. Boston: Beacon.
Freud, S. (1910). The origin and development of psychoanalysis. *American Journal of Psychology*, *21*(2), 181–218. doi: 10.2307/1413001.
Kalayjian, A. (2002). Biopsychosocial and spiritual treatment of trauma. In R. Massey & S Massey (eds.), *Comprehensive handbook of psychotherapy*, vol. 3 (pp. 615–37). New York: John Wiley & Sons.
Kalayjian, A. (2015). *Seven-step integrative healing model: Biopsychosocial and ecospiritual model for healing, transforming disputes, conflict transformation, peace building, and forgiveness*. Retrieved fromhttp://meaningfulworld.com/wp-content/uploads/2015/08/7-Step-Integrative-Healing-Model-by-Dr-Kalayjian-2015.pdf.
Kalayjian, A., & Eugene, D. (eds.). (2010a). *Mass trauma and emotional healing around the world: Rituals and practices for resilience and meaning-making*, vol. 1. Santa Barbara, CA: ABC-CLIO.
Kalayjian, A., & Eugene, D. (eds.). (2010b). *Mass trauma and emotional healing around the world: Rituals and practices for resilience and meaning-making*, vol. 2. Santa Barbara, CA: ABC-CLIO.
Kalayjian, A., & Paloutzian, R. (2010). *Forgiveness and reconciliation: Psychological pathways to conflict transformation and peace building*. New York: Springer.
Kalayjian, A., Shigemoto, Y., & Patel, B. (2010). Earthquake in Soviet Armenia: Coping, integration, and meaning-making. In A. Kalayjian & D. Eugene (eds.), *Mass trauma and emotional healing around the world: Rituals and practices for resilience and meaning-making*, vol. 1 (pp. 1–21). Santa Barbara, CA: ABC-CLIO.
Kalayjian, A., & Sofletea, G. (2012). Case study from Sierra Leone. In S. Poyrazli & C. Thompson (eds.), *International case studies in mental health* (pp. 33–51). Thousand Oaks, CA: Sage.
Kleijn, W. C., Hovens, J. E., & Rodenburg, J. J. (2001). Posttraumatic stress symptoms in refugees: Assessments with the Harvard Trauma Questionnaire and the Hopkins Symptom Checklist-25 in different languages. *Psychological Reports*, *88*(2), 527–32. doi: 10.2466/PR0.88.2.527-532.
Roxberg, Å., Burman, M., Guldbrand, M., Fridlund, B., & Barbosa da Silva, A. (2010). Out of the wave: The meaning of suffering and relieved suffering for survivors of the tsunami catastrophe. A hermeneutic-phenomenological study of TV interviews one year after the tsunami catastrophe, 2004. *Scandinavian Journal of Caring Sciences*, *24*(4), 707–15. doi: 10.1111/j.1471-6712.2009.00767.x.
Skaggs, B. G., & Barron, C. R. (2006). Searching for meaning in negative events: Concept analysis. *Journal of Advanced Nursing*, *53*, 559–70.
Steger, M. F., Frazier, P., Oishi, S., & Kaler, M. (2006). The Meaning in Life Questionnaire: Assessing the presence of and search for meaning in life. *Journal of Counseling Psychology*, *53*(1), 80–93. doi: 10.1037/0022-0167.53.1.80.
Sullivan, H. S. (1953). The interpersonal theory of psychiatry. New York: W. W. Norton.
Toussaint, L. L., Kalayjian, A., & Diakonova-Curtis, D. (2017). Forgiveness makes sense: Forgiving others enhances the salutary associations of meaning-making with traumatic stress symptoms. *Peace and Conflict: Journal of Peace Psychology*, *23*(1), 85–88.
Toussaint, L. L., Kalayjian, A., Herman, K., Hein, A., Maseko, N., & Diakonova-Curtis, D. (2017). Traumatic stress symptoms, forgiveness, and meaning in life in four traumatized regions of the world. *International Perspectives in Psychology: Research, Practice, Consultation*, *6*(1), 5.
Van der Kolk, B. A. (1987). The drug treatment of posttraumatic stress disorder. *Journal of Affective Disorders*, *13*(2), 203–13.

Van der Kolk, B. A., & Saporta, L. (1993). Biological response to psychic trauma. In J. P. Wilson & B. Raphael (eds.), *International handbook of traumatic stress syndromes* (pp. 25–33). New York: Plenum.

Chapter Four

Expressive Art for Helping Children Heal in Crisis and Disaster

Judy Kuriansky

Natural disasters, as well as other crises, like epidemics, have been numerous in the past few decades, affecting areas throughout the world, claiming thousands of lives and destroying property and livelihoods. These non-man-made disasters include earthquakes, floods, tsunamis, and fires, as well as outbreaks of health viral disease. My own extensive experience, as well as that of others, has shown that the immediate and long-term psychological impacts of such events affect those both directly and indirectly impacted (Chan et al., 2016; Kuriansky, 2013b, 2015, 2016a, 2016c; Kuriansky, Wu et al., 2015).

Research, which has shown that the impacts on children can be vast, has also demonstrated the usefulness of artistic techniques to aid in their recovery (Laor et al., 2002; La Greca et al., 2002). While "therapy" itself has cultural taboos in various settings, art is a universal, nonthreatening activity that has underlying therapeutic gains and is a common activity generally experienced as play by children. Creating and reflecting on one's works of art increases awareness of self and connection with others, aids in coping with stress and traumatic experiences, and affirms life and pleasure (American Art Therapy Association, n.d.). Arts activities have been shown to be an effective language-independent medium to heal children from trauma, including tsunamis, by nurturing their creativity and connecting them to others (International Child Art Foundation, n.d.). Many international organizations have used varieties of art activities to help children heal from traumatic situations, for example, the Red Cross and Red Crescent Societies, and Save the Children.

This paper traces my experience in applying selected techniques of art therapy in interventions throughout the world during a period of several decades, using a combination of exercises from my toolbox of psychosocial and psychoeducational techniques, designed to help children heal from natural disasters and other crises, for instance, epidemics, in various cultures and settings (Kuriansky, 2008). The art activities reported in this chapter focus specifically on drawing exercises, as well as making artistic constructions, in the context of other techniques that were also applied. The interventions were done with groups, most of which (when time and circumstances allowed) were conducted in the form of trainings in a train-the-trainers three-tier model, whereby the master trainer trained adult trainees, who then directed the workshop with children (Kuriansky, Margevich et al., 2017). Different teams participated with me in each intervention, as warranted by the circumstances and/or immediacy of the disaster. The value of such approaches for children is described and highlighted here as adaptable to different circumstances.

The workshops are consistent with the basic level of the Inter-Agency Standing Committee (IASC) guidelines, in providing fundamental psychosocial support and well-being to a broad group. They are not meant to address more complicated trauma symptoms that require more focused support and specialized services.

CONCEPTUAL FRAMEWORK

The art techniques described in this chapter are based on sound principles in the field of stress, traumatology, and psychosocial resilience, including in disaster preparation, risk recovery postdisaster, and reintegration. The key principles include (although they are not limited to) the following:

- Children are generally resilient but need, and respond well to, psychosocial intervention postdisaster, especially as the impact of such traumas can be long-lasting.
- Children (as well as people of all ages) who have been through a trauma benefit from knowing that they are not alone and that others (including service providers and peers, and even those far away who have experienced similar traumas) support and care about them.
- Children posttrauma respond well to recreational projects, especially those including art activities, which may be mixed with other techniques, like music, dance, and play.
- Simple techniques tend to have deeper psychological meaning and healing properties that can be experienced by children with easy-to-understand lessons; these have psychological impact but do not require "deep" processing, although explanations and discussion of the purpose and intended outcome of the exercises are certainly valuable.

- Artistic techniques can, of course, be applied by experienced therapists, but also by volunteers and community individuals following simple instruction (Kuriansky, Zinsou et al., 2015).
- An overriding goal is to instill hope to counteract the deep sense of loss and hopelessness that the trauma has created.

The artistic techniques in the interventions were aimed at these three "gold standard" psychological constructs: resilience, empowerment, and connection to others. The usefulness of these constructs in aiding recovery has been described and used as a focus for many interventions on my part. Key to achieving them in times of disaster and tragedy is the establishment of safety; therefore, where possible, participants were asked to draw in a safe space (Kuriansky, 2018; Kuriansky, Polizer, & Zinsou, 2016).

The following definition of *resilience* is a biopsychosocial and spiritual response that reflects the "ability to bounce back from a crisis, to engage in positive coping actions, to request and accept support, and to look forward toward a better future" (Nemeth & Olivier, 2017). *Empowerment* is a theoretical model for understanding the process and consequences of efforts to exert control and influence over decisions and actions that affect one's life personally, to achieve self-efficacy, and to work as a community (Berry et al., 2013; Zimmerman, 2000). The value of social cohesion is well documented, whereby sharing, engagement, and common purpose build resilience (Rodin, 2014).

The two art activities aimed at achieving these states that are focused on in this chapter are projective drawings and art construction. The projective drawings activity involved variations according to the needs and logistics of the setting and the particular workshop plan (e.g., timing, agreement with partners, consistency with the other activities). These included drawing a family, the incident, the bridge drawing, and a safe space, as shown in figure 4.1. This activity, as noted earlier, was incorporated into other activities—for example, after drawing a safe space, participants were asked to find a place in the room that felt safe and to elaborate on what about it felt safe, as well as who in their life helped them feel safe, and to post their drawings on the wall and share about them.

The bridge drawing was originally designed as a projective assessment in which individuals generate an image that is thought to reflect their perceptions of their past, present, and future life; drawing a bridge "from someplace to someplace" displays elements of an individual's perceptions of life movement, transition, conflicts, and barriers (Hays & Lyons, 1981). Later research identified four coping styles to aid in the diagnosis and treatment of problems in children: repressors, suppressors, synthesizers, and sensitizers. Depending on the stability of the bridge and the self, and the danger of the surroundings, these styles indicated more or less need for support or therapy (Yedida &

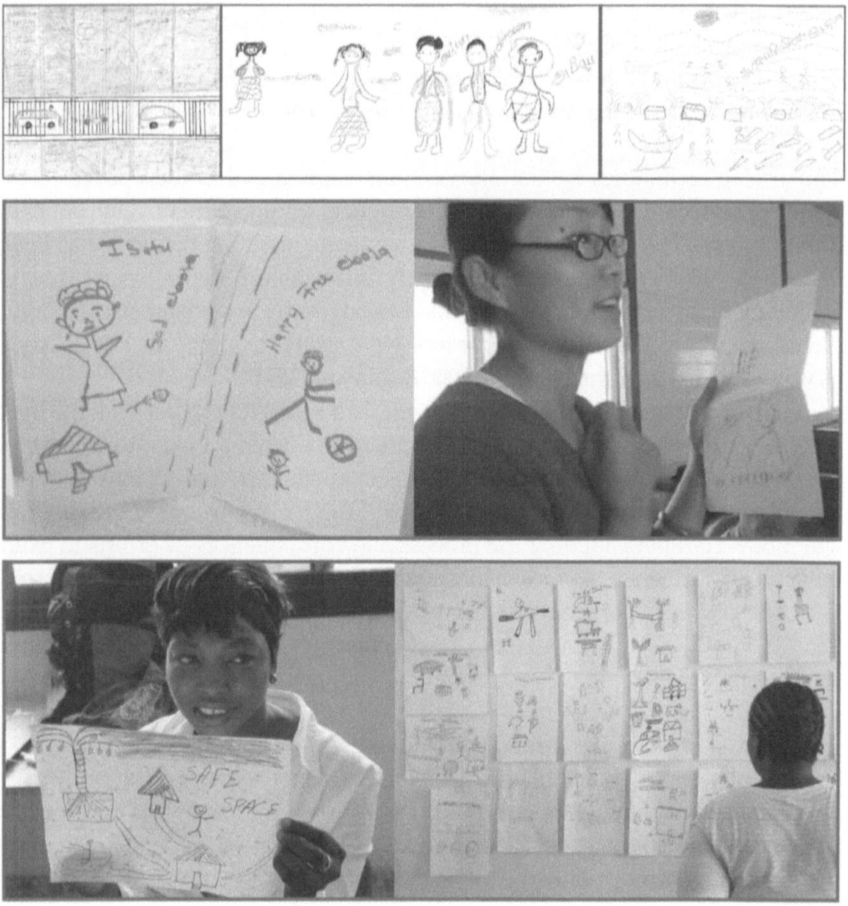

Figure 4.1. (Top): Sri Lanka child drawings posttsunami of bridge, family, and the trauma; (center): bridge drawings by participant in Sierra Leone during Ebola workshop and by teacher in China postearthquake training; (bottom): safe space drawings by youth in Sierra Leone during Ebola workshop and by the group. ***Judy Kuriansky***

Itzahaky, 2004). The present variation was simpler. Applicable to these situations, it involved instructions to draw the trauma on the left side of the page and a happier experience on the opposite (right) side, with a bridge on the paper fold as a way to transition from the trauma to greater happiness.

The art construction activity has evolved during various missions, from designing on a form, to constructing a culturally relevant object, to the ultimately constructive activity of designing with Sharpie colored pens on one side of a small soft (felt) rectangle, then folded over to be sewn into the shape of a pillow, as shown in figure 4.2.

The activity is meant to be experienced as play (with oneself and/or others), as projective expression, and as enabling contact comfort, to be cuddled and slept with. It can also be considered a "transitional object" (like the traditional teddy bear), symbolizing the parental/maternal nurturing figure and providing security for emotional support. Developed by myself, this iteration has been combined with additional activities, for instance, exchanges with other children throughout the world who have also carried out the activity, to achieve the psychological advantages of knowing they are not the only one who has suffered, becoming aware that other children care, and achieving connection with others in the immediate and global community.

Children should draw on the material and make it into a pillow. They can draw a bird and add anything they want, like their name and any message

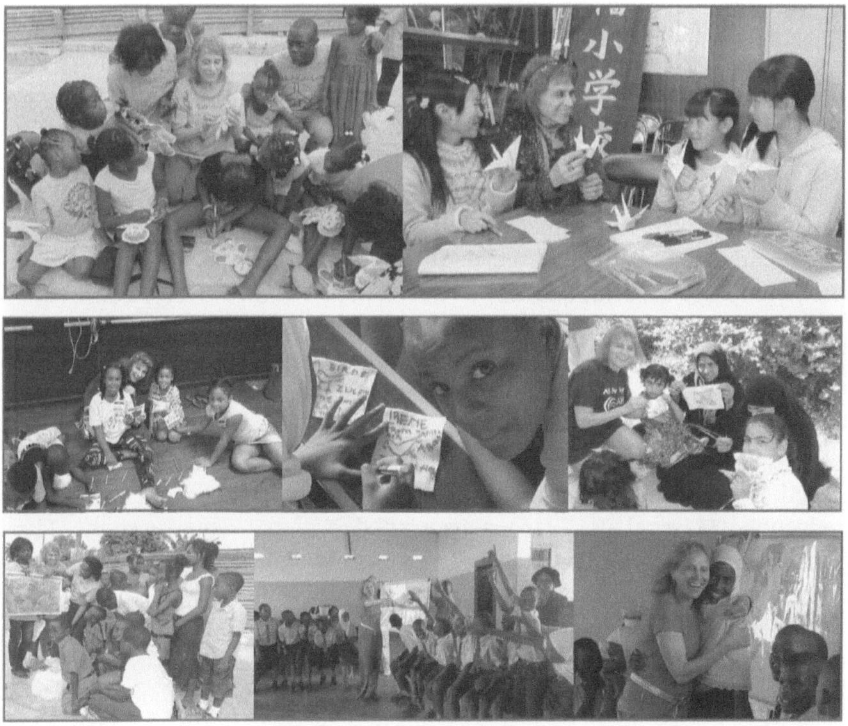

Figure 4.2. (Top): Art object construction in Haiti and Japan postearthquake workshops; (center): pillow construction in St. Maarten, Tanzania, and Jordan workshops; (bottom): geography lesson with Haiti and Tanzania youth. *Judy Kuriansky*

they would like to send to another child about their experience or their home. They can draw a bird because birds fly to other places easily, so they can bring messages easily and connect one person to others.

Depending on the situation, participants should be told that they can keep their pillows (to feel good or to play with) or that they will be collected to be sent to another child who has had similar experiences, in which case they are given a pillow made by a child from another country.

The activity works well when combined with a geography lesson, drawing children's attention to a large map of the world posted on the wall. Other countries where children have experienced similar traumas should be described, and children should be invited to come up and show where those countries are located, with elaborated discussion regarding how far away they are, what happened there, and how the children are coping. When constructions that were made by participants in another country are available for exchange, the location and events in those countries can be discussed. Crayons (washable for vinyl maps) can be used to trace the routes between countries.

These techniques have been integrated into training workshops through various combinations of activities from my toolbox. Many of them are continually developed; chosen to be consistent with the logistics and needs of the particular population; and aimed at increasing local capacity, especially in low-resource conditions and settings. I developed the format and content with input from the other partners in the various settings; some were also codeveloped with my project partner and international musician, Russell Daisey, in the Global Kids Connect Project, whose components include simple psychological techniques for stress reduction and recovery, construction (with exchange and a geography lesson, when possible) of an object with a message of hope, and cultural programming. The interventions have been described in many articles in professional journals and at many international conferences.

Presentations and demonstrations have been made at many international psychological conferences and at United Nations meetings about disaster risk reduction (Masangkay, 2015). One United Nations venue was the Third World Conference on Disaster Risk Reduction—From Commitment to Action, held in Sendai, Japan, in March 2015, where I, with colleague Father Wismick Jean-Charles and interns Joel Zinsou and Quyen Nguyen, conducted several workshops at the youth conference organized by the United Nations Major Group for Children and Youth. Another was the Global Platform for Disaster Risk Reduction, held in Cancún, Mexico, in May 2017, where I and a student assistant, Aleandra Marevich, led demonstrations of the object construction procedure for attendees at the visitor exhibit booth run by the United Nations Major Group for Children and Youth. Participants from

European and South American countries (e.g., Peru) expressed great interest in applying the object construction activity in their own contexts.

Furthermore, the activities are consistent with theories of the value of expressive arts, whereby children can express themselves without judgment or criticism in a safe and accepting environment, playing out events or alternate paths and different endings to make sense of events or experience the world in a different way, managing difficult experiences, as well as connecting them with their inner selves and simultaneously with the group, the community, and the world (Malchiodi, 2005; Smilan, 2009).

The interventions are consistent with two important international documents calling for psychosocial recovery. The first is the United Nations 2030 Agenda for Sustainable Development, which includes a historical target to "promote mental health and well-being" (United Nations, 2015), for which I negotiated in partnership with the ambassador of the Republic of Palau to the United Nations, public health physician Dr. Caleb Otto (Forman, 2014; Kuriansky, 2018, 2016b). The second is the Sendai Framework for Disaster Risk Reduction 2015–2030, paragraph 33 90, which states the goal to "enhance recovery schemes to provide psychosocial support and mental health services for all people in need" (UNISDR, 2015).

APPLICATIONS IN VARIOUS CULTURES AND SETTINGS

Haiti

A devastating earthquake of magnitude 7.0 struck Haiti on the afternoon of January 12, 2010, as yet another disaster in a small country that had suffered previous natural disasters, as well as decades of social, economic, and political problems, inequalities, and a severely inadequate and fractured mental health system. In that tragedy, in the areas surrounding the capital city of Port-au-Prince, 230,000 people lost their lives, and more than 70 percent of homes were damaged. My commitment to the country had begun in partnership with Father Wismick Jean-Charles, a Haitian Catholic priest who I recruited as a representative of the International Association of Applied Psychology, a United Nations ECOSOC-accredited NGO of which I am a main representative. We had traveled to Jean-Charles's hometown to promote development, poverty reduction, and community services for children, participating in projects to achieve rapport between Haitian and Dominican Republic youth, e.g., through FUNGLODE (the United Nations Association of the Dominican Republic) and Haitian Action for the United Nations. Immediately after the January 2010 earthquake we went to Haiti to provide emergency psychosocial support, training students and volunteers to provide assistance at Father Jean-Charles's St. Louis de Roi church community and at a local hospital, L'Hôpital de la Communauté Haïtienne.

Many subsequent preplanned missions provided trainings for students and community volunteers using my toolbox, intended for postrecovery of that disaster and also after devastating Hurricane Matthew in October 2016 (Kuriansky, 2010a, 2010b, 2017; Kuriansky & Jean-Charles, 2012). These included various implementations of the object construction and geography lesson, as shown in figure 4.2. The project began with construction in muslin of a doll-figure stuffed with cotton and decorated with colored pens, based on a collaboration with a Japanese-based NGO called "Happy Doll." It evolved into the subsequently widely used pillow form, which proved to be more practical, given the simplicity of the shape and ease of construction.

I assisted Jean-Charles in founding the first mental health support center in Haiti, called CESSA, a French acronym for Centre de Spiritualité, d'Evangélisation, et de Santé Mentale, which refers to spirituality and mental health (Jean-Charles, 2011a, 2011b). It was planned to train and empower local leaders, clergy members, young professionals, and teachers and students through partnerships, and to develop best-practice interventions that were culturally appropriate and sustainable.

Research with local Haitian volunteer helpers and trainees in my workshops, with quantitative responses to pre- and postquestionnaires, and qualitative responses, showed positive results, including participants' reports of increased interest, confidence, and skill in working with children, as well as feeling better about themselves and more empowered (Kuriansky, Margevich et al., 2017).

A training was held in September 2011, at St. Luke's Hospital in New York City, on the 10th anniversary of the 9-11 terrorist attacks on the World Trade Center, for children in the outpatient department of the hospital. This represented an application of the techniques in the context of recovery from a man-made tragedy; while not the focus of this chapter, it was interesting to note similarities in usefulness in such a different context (Kuriansky, 2013d).

Japan

The earthquake/tsunami in Japan took place on March 11, 2011, centered in Sendai, with the added explosion of the nearby nuclear power plant in Fukushima; the disaster resulted in almost 16,000 deaths and the massive destruction of homes. The first postevent visit to Japan involved me, along with my project partner and international musician Russell Daisey, attending the "Songs of Hope" concert in October 2011, in Hakuju Hall in Tokyo, featuring opera singer Tomoko Shibata; it was an opportunity to take advantage of the opportunity to assist children and improvise workshop activities.

The concept of children drawing on an item that can include a message and then be exchanged with children in other locations was used to show commonality, solidarity, and shared experiences. In an early version of the construction activity, cardboard cutout figures of people and of hearts, along with colored pens (purchased from an arts store in New York) were handed out to children who were brought by partners collaborating in the event. These constructions were given to Haiti children in a subsequent mission to that country, to show solidarity between the victims of earthquakes or tsunamis in both locations.

The next mission was held on the first anniversary of the tsunami/earthquake, in March 2012, in Sendai, Japan, in partnership with a local nonprofit organization, the Recovery Assistance Program of Miyagi (Gambaro Miyagi) (Kuriansky, 2011a, 2012b, 2012c). These resulted from a meeting of the partners at an event at the United Nations related to the tsunami and carried out a week later. Workshops were held in three schools in the area, including in some small groups where cranes were made, and in some large auditoriums with hundreds of children, where many activities were carried out, including the pillow construction. Due to time and logistical considerations, in one large auditorium, while the children were doing other activities, the mothers sitting in the back of the room constructed the origami cranes, then inscribed with messages. This experience, which demonstrated the implementation of the activity adjusted for the logistics of the situation, led to the valuable element of involving parents in the construction. This was implemented in a more formal way in Haiti and Jordan (described later in this chapter), where mothers were recruited to sew the pillows after the children had drawn on them.

An event on May 20, 2012, featured my presentation of the mission, a demonstration of the cranes constructed by the children, along with additional cranes made for future distribution, and other expressive activities (performances of music by Russell Daisey and dance by the Yuko Takahashi Dance Company from Miyagi). Also displayed was an original 30-foot artistic scroll by Jave Yoshimoto, demonstrating the stages of trauma and recovery, called "Baptism of Concrete Estuary." The event was held in New York City at the famed Art Students League to benefit the Music and Art without Borders program of Gambaro Miyagi and the Art Students League scholarship program.

Sierra Leone

The West African Ebola virus epidemic of 2014 was the geographically widest outbreak of that disease in history, causing major loss of life and socioeconomic disruption in the region, mainly in the countries of Guinea, Liberia, and Sierra Leone. I went to Sierra Leone during the outbreak to provide psychosocial trainings, in partnership with other international aid organizations and groups on the ground (Cohen, 2015; Kuriansky, 2017; Kuriansky, Polizer, & Zinsou, 2016).

My trainings (Kuriansky, Polizer, & Zinsou, 2016), in partnership with IsraAid, Caritas, and UNICEF, were conducted with community volunteers, who subsequently led the workshop with children at the Community Center in Hastings, a town about 15 miles east of the capital city of Freetown. A training was also carried out with the staff of the Sierra Leone Child Welfare Society. Both settings included the bridge drawing, but the first setting, held during the course of five days, included more drawings. Especially significant were the children's drawings of a safe space, as shown in figure 4.1. These were posted on the wall for the group to observe and discuss.

In the Hastings Community Center training, the bridge drawing by a male participant, Isatu (shown in figure 4.1), shows post-Ebola sadness (i.e., he wrote the word "sad" and drew a mother crying, with a figure lying down, identified as a family member succumbing to the virus). The Ebola-free conditions on the opposite side of the page show the contrasting word "happy" and two males playing soccer. The bridge lines are broken up, which is consistent with the fact that the Ebola-free condition had not yet happened; however, some optimism is evident in the three lines outlined for the bridge.

The participants also constructed the pillows, many of which, despite the dire reality of the Ebola outbreak, displayed sunshine, hearts, and greenery, also suggesting optimism, as shown in figure 4.2.

These applications demonstrate positive outcomes, shown in preliminary research, as well as in unstructured reports by the trainees and observations by the master trainers. They further confirm the success of application of these techniques in situations characterized by the effects of an epidemic, as well as those of natural disasters (Kuriansky et al., 2017).

Sint Maarten

A training workshop for teachers and allied professionals was conducted in Sint Maarten on the anniversary of Hurricane Irma. The "Mission for Well-being and Psychosocial Recovery Post-Hurricane in Sint Maarten" was a collaboration between my team members from the International Association of Applied Psychology and allied colleagues (e.g., yoga expert Cathleen deKerchove) with the Art Saves Lives Foundation and the St. Maarten National Institutes for the Arts-St. Maarten, supported by the Department of Culture of the Government of Sint Maarten, headed by Clara Reyes. The five-day training involved the pillow construction (shown in figure 4.2), as well as several other activities from the toolbox.

Preliminary analysis of a questionnaire administered to the trainees about their experience revealed that, similar to the results for the trainings in Sierra Leone, participants reported both personal and professional gains from the experience. In unstructured questioning, several trainees mentioned immediately putting the techniques to use with the children with whom they worked.

They also were impressed with the children's enthusiastic responses to the pillow construction activity, combined with the geography lesson. In the training, the children were observed to be totally absorbed in looking at the map mounted on the wall and discussing the questions about countries where children had experienced traumas similar to their own. One child eagerly pointed out where Japan was located, explained what a tsunami was, and then observed that those children "had more water than me."

Louisiana

An extremely destructive and deadly category 5 hurricane made landfall in August 2005, on Florida and Louisiana, particularly the city of New Orleans and surrounding areas, causing catastrophic damage from Central Florida to eastern Texas. In its wake, Hurricane Katrina left much physical damage and emotional trauma.

Consistent with recommendations based on research about the long-term emotional effects of trauma, anniversary wellness workshops were held in New Orleans on the first and 10th anniversaries of the disaster, organized by noted Louisiana neuropsychologist Dr. Darlyne Nemeth, supported by the Louisiana Psychological Association and endorsed by the World Council for Psychotherapy (Nemeth, 2018). The Anniversary Wellness and Emotional Resiliency workshops included basic information about trauma, as well as group activities led by Nemeth and me, including relaxation exercises, community cohesion exercises, anxiety-reduction techniques, expressions of appreciation, and creative construction activities. A comparison of pre- and postresearch showed a reduction of anxiety levels and increasing resilience as measured by various scales. It was observed that the Louisiana children enjoyed preparing pillows for others, even as the Haitian children had prepared pillows for them (Kuriansky, 2012a; Nemeth, 2018; Nemeth, Kuriansky, Olivier et al., 2012; Nemeth, Kuriansky, Reeder et al., 2011; Peveto, 2016).

In August 2016, severe flooding inundated Baton Rouge, Louisiana, causing emotional trauma and retriggering, in some cases, emotional reactions felt only four months earlier in March 2016, as well as during Hurricane Katrina in 2005. As a result, Nemeth and I conducted another workshop on December 3, 2016, with members of the Florida Boulevard Baptist Church. Nemeth described principles of trauma and resilience, while I demonstrated various activities from the toolbox, while focusing the time allotted on the pillow construction with extended discussion of the experience of doing the activity, as well as the emotions it aroused. The small size of the group allowed for an intensive discussion about personal coping, as well as training of the attendees to apply the technique with children of the church community.

One woman, after describing her bird drawing, elaborated on her experience of other traumas, including her present difficulties with her father's condition. This demonstrated how applicable the technique is to adults, even as they are learning how to lead the experience with children, and also how the simple, outwardly fun activity can open the door to a much deeper conversation. The woman expressed great appreciation for having been able to share her experience, especially with a trained psychologist.

Tanzania

A workshop was conducted at the Royal School in Arusha, Tanzania, with children, all of whom were living in poverty, and some of whom were abandoned or orphaned. Suitable techniques were chosen from my toolbox, given the large number of children in a large space. These included the pillow construction, with the children drawing birds and messages, as shown in figure 4.2.

For the exchange, given the large numbers, the children were given origami cranes made by children in Japan. The children participating in the geography lesson showed great eagerness (as in other cultures), rushing to the world map, enthusiastically searching for Japan, and appearing delighted to discover the location and guess how far (in miles or hours) the children in Japan were from them in Africa, as shown in figure 4.2.

The teacher reported, "It went very well . . . the children got a chance to feel good."

Jordan

As a result of the war in Syria, many refugees have sought haven in Jordan, where they live in difficult conditions. I participated in a medical and humanitarian mission to Amman, Jordan, in October 2016, to assist people in need of medical services, including (but not limited to) displaced Syrians in Jordan. The mission was organized by a small Massachusetts-based nonprofit, Atlantic Humanitarian Relief, led by Dr. Humam Akbik, MD, a Cincinnati-based anesthesiologist and pain management specialist. The group consisted of dozens of medical volunteers from throughout the world; three psychosocial volunteers (myself, a psychologist from California, and a psychiatry resident from the United Kingdom who was an Arabic-speaking student of mine); and about 20 other volunteers who provided support (packing supplies, organizing teams, etc.). Community members came to clinics outside the capital city of Amman, bringing their children.

I conducted trainings of team members with a combination of techniques from her toolbox, including the pillow construction, that were deemed appropriate for the culture and were then conducted with a group of children.

Particularly important was involving the mothers to sew the pillows, as shown in figure 4.2, to build on the cultural family bonding.

My student, who returned the next year with the same group, repeated the trainings and activities in school settings. Positive outcomes were reported in terms of the receptivity of the students and teachers, and considerable satisfaction with the intervention.

China

A major earthquake measuring 7.1 on the Richter scale hit the isolated high-altitude Yushu Tibetan Autonomous Prefecture in Qinghai province, China, on April 14, 2010, leaving about 2,700 dead and more than 12,000 injured, with 15,000 collapsed homes and about 100,000 people homeless, then living in tents. More than 11 schools were destroyed.

I went on a mission to the earthquake site with Chinese colleagues from the International Association of Chinese Medical Specialists and Psychologists, led by Dr. Mingyu Deng, to conduct workshops for children in several surviving schools and trainings for teachers to help children cope. In the teacher training, I instructed participants about how to use the bridge drawing to reassure the children that they can go from an unhappy place to a happy place with their inner power and the power of their minds. One teacher, shown in figure 4.1, who shared with the group about her drawing, described that one side showed, "I am very sad, crying," but the bridge showed "going through to the mountains and the sun." In response to the question, "How do you feel?" she declared, "I feel better."

Sri Lanka

The Indian Ocean earthquake and tsunami that struck on December 26, 2004, caused severe destruction and the deaths of about 230,000 people, including about 30,000 in Sri Lanka, of whom 12,000 were children. More than 900 children were orphaned, and many others lost family members. I participated in a healing mission to Batticaloa, the northeastern coast of Sri Lanka, five weeks after the disaster, as part of a disaster relief project training professional volunteers and local psychosocial facilitators organized by the Association for Disaster and Mass Trauma Studies. To complicate matters, this area of the country had been hard hit by civil war, which had wreaked havoc on the lives of the population for almost 20 years and resulted in additional practical and emotional burdens.

The children who received the intervention were living in temporary shelters at the time, with the property destruction visible everywhere a constant reminder of their extensive losses. Many were experiencing a variety of fears resulting from trauma, stress, grief, bereavement, and depression. At the same time, they were able to express joy and playfulness appropriately, demonstrating their culturally derived and socially reinforced resilience. While much has been written on the use of intervention strategies with children in cases of trauma arising from such stressors as sexual abuse, illness, and violence, few studies have addressed the efficacy of intervention strategies as a result of natural disasters. This discussion is an attempt to improve documentation and support for this approach with children in these circumstances.

More than 70 children participated in my various groups, which were intended to reduce fears and nightmares, and reinforce coping skills and mastery. The art techniques included drawing pictures and telling the story of their families and the tsunami, as well as techniques like reframing nightmares of family members' deaths, in vivo desensitization of fears of the sea as the site of deaths, breathing and safety techniques, safety exercises, memorial rituals, and other activities in my toolbox (Kuriansky, 2008). Children anecdotally reported a notable decrease in fears and demonstrated improvement in mood.

The sessions were held for a group of children in a classroom on the grounds of a college where emergency housing was also provided. Children were asked to do the bridge drawing and then share what they had drawn. Their depictions of their families and the tsunami, which they had also been asked to include, gave added insight into interpreting their situations and capacity to cope by analyzing which people were in the drawing and who was missing (e.g., who had died in the tsunami), consistent with the draw-a-family exercise (Biasi, Bonaiuto, & Levin, 2015). As the children spoke in the Tamil language, an interpreter was used, a local young male volunteer who spoke English well. I interpreted the three drawings together, based on years of such experiences. To process exercise for the purpose of healing, the children were then engaged in a discussion aimed at building self-esteem and hopes for the future, including the idea that family members who had been lost would want the child to live on with hope. These themes were based on extensive professional experience and indicators from past research of these drawing exercises. For example, the question was asked, "What is a quality about you that your parent was proud of?" Then the other children were asked to repeat back that quality to the child, to have the child experience validation and enhanced self-esteem.

The Case of Vidya

The bridge drawing of this 12-year-old girl was very defined and organized, with constructed lines that seemed to contain more chaotic drawing underneath. Some figures appeared vaguely at the bottom (a possible indication of the child's losses and distress), while a heart emerged from the bridge to the upper part of the drawing, indicating hope. The bridge itself was drawn in black marker, with cars clearly crossing over it to the other side, a design that could be interpreted as symbolic of her degree of coping. The three cars were all different shapes and sizes. Colorful lines extended through the bridge and over the lagoon, suggesting greater protection and a grasp on keeping herself stable, along with containment of her emotions and movement through the disaster, indicating some inner strength to overcome trauma.

In fact, her experience during the tsunami was tragic. While she survived by climbing a tree, other family members perished. Vidya's drawing of her family showed her mother, brother, and father on one side, while she and her sister were on the other side. The figures were rounded, with distinct black hair. Her father's head was circled lightly. She related that her mother, brother, and sister were in a small boat that capsized during the tsunami, and that her brother was the only survivor. She stated, "I couldn't help my mother and sister; I lost them." She spoke of having nightmares where she heard screaming, and where she was running away from the water and the waves.

In discussion, when I focused on what qualities her mother and sister would appreciate in her, she responded that she was clever and pretty. When these words were repeated back to her, she smiled and asked to be hugged. Her drawing of the tsunami showed the boat, with her mother, brother, and sister inside, that had capsized. Many other people and logs are at the bottom, presumably in danger comparable to her family in the boat. Yet, the houses were defined, and, as in her bridge drawing, there was structure to the composition. Wavy lines might indicate that all was submerged, but not very clearly. While the day was, in reality, sunny, the presence of the sun shining and smiling could be interpreted as consistent with her bridge drawing as indicating a capacity for emotional regulation and dealing with her intense loss.

Applying the techniques described here, whereby the child announces a quality of which the parent would be proud, Vidya said that her mother (who perished in the boat) would have said, "You are clever" (for climbing a tree to survive). After three other children repeated, "Vidya, you are clever," I elaborated on this, complimenting Vidya's ability to find solutions in the most difficult conditions and noting how that presaged well for her future.

DISCUSSION AND CONCLUSIONS

The various activities in these trainings can be seen as addressing the basic principles of art and play therapy, along with the constructs of resilience, empowerment, and connection. The two activities that my colleagues and I implemented, as described in this chapter, have been widely accepted and enjoyed in many contexts across many cultures, overcoming language barriers and being universally experienced as fun. Moreover, it is relatively easy to train volunteers and paraprofessionals to use them, thereby increasing capacity, especially in low-resource settings following disasters.

The object construction activity, in particular, generates a great deal of engagement and even glee on the part of the children. This activity can be a full workshop of its own, without being combined with other activities, allowing more time to draw, exchange products, and share the experience.

Certain guidelines are useful when incorporating these activities into a workshop. These include giving instructions to the trainees about the implications and psychological foundations for the activities so that they understand them, while at the same time noting that these do not have to be communicated to the children, who can just enjoy the activities. By the same token, trainees can improvise and, depending on the receptivity of the children, develop deeper discussions about the activity, and explore "lessons learned," by gently asking the children more probing questions, for example, "How do you feel about what you created?" "What feelings do you have that you would like to share?" "What does this experience remind you of?" "What would you like to share with the other children about what you did?" Experiences can be shared by partnering children with others or inviting them to convey them to the group.

Improvisation is key when thinking of needed materials or ways to adapt exercises, for example, in remote villages. Thus, if paper is not available for the drawing exercises, leaders might have participants create a construction using materials from the environment (e.g., stones, sticks, and leaves). Also, for the pillow exercise, local material (e.g., muslin) can be purchased, but, if it is not available or costly, leaders need to think outside the box to create a new idea (even if the product cannot then be shared), like making a bird shape on the ground using palm fronds as wings; alternatively, if paper is available, the children can draw a bird and write a message on it.

End products can be kept, exchanged with other children in the group or in neighboring communities, or given to the leaders for children in other countries, if they are receiving a product from another country. Involving parents in the activities aimed for the children aids in fostering parent–child closeness and bonding, while concluding the workshop experience with a group exercise is preferable for closure and connection. This can be a song; I use "Hope Is Alive," a song composed by myself and my project collaborator, Russell Daisey.

While the activities described here are very nonthreatening, the trainer/workshop leader should always be on the alert for any child who seems to be having problems, whether mild difficulties in understanding or following the exercises, or more serious emotional issues (evident in symptoms like withdrawal, a sad-looking face, or being grumpy or overly assertive with others).

In general, adults respond well to these activities. Research has shown that trainees learn a great deal about how to help children cope and feel comfortable about the process; they also grow personally, as well as professionally (Kuriansky, Zinsou et al., 2015). Adult trainees also self-report having had fun, learned about themselves, and processed their own trauma; moreover, team leaders and I have observed them doing so.

While some research has been conducted and reported about the experiences of trainers leading these activities with children, little has been completed about the impact of these experiences on the children themselves. While a structured self-report evaluation has been repeatedly planned in the various settings described in this chapter, using appropriate measuring scales for children—e.g., facial expressions—it has not been possible to carry them out due to lack of time after the workshop itself was completed or other commitments for the children (e.g., to be bussed back to their homes or communities).

The experiences described in this chapter show the value of such interventions for recovery, along with advocacy for artistic psychoeducational techniques in disaster recovery (Kuriansky, 2011b). They further demonstrate the value of applying these particular art activities in diverse cultures, while calling for further research to validate their effectiveness as evidence-based interventions to help children cope in various crises, including natural disasters and epidemics.

ACKNOWLEDGMENTS

The following people participated in different ways in various projects described in this paper: Russell Daisey, Father Wismick Jean-Charles, Dr. Alexandra Margevich, Dr. Darlyne Nemeth, Yotam Polizer, Dr. Miller Deng, Megan Leduc, Ann Flynn, Marina Masic, Cathleen deKerchove, and Michelin Aboukasm.

REFERENCES

American Art Therapy Association. (n.d.). Retrieved from https://arttherapy.org.

Berry, M. O., Kuriansky, J., Lytle, M., & Vistman, B. (2013, December). Entrepreneurial training for girls empowerment in Lesotho: A process evaluation of a model programme. *South African Journal of Psychology*, *43*(4), 446–58.

Biasi, V., Bonaiuto, P., & Levin, J. M. (2015). The "Colour Family Drawing Test": Assessing children's perception of family relationships. Studies on Mental Health and Cross-Cultural Comparisons. *Health*, *7*, 300–7. Retrieved from http://www.scirp.org/journal/health.

Chan, K. L., Chau, W. W., Kuriansky, J., Dow, E., Zinsou, J. C., Leung, J., & Kim, S. (2016). The psychosocial and interpersonal impact of the SARS epidemic on Chinese health professionals: Implications for epidemics, including Ebola. In J. Kuriansky (ed.), *The psychosocial aspects of a deadly epidemic: What Ebola has taught us about holistic healing* (pp. 287–321). Santa Barbara, CA: ABC-CLIO/Praeger.

Cohen, B. (2015, February). How a New York psychologist and an Israeli humanitarian organization are helping Sierra Leone stand up to Ebola. *Algemeiner*. Retrieved from http://www.

algemeiner.com/2015/02/09/how-a-new-york-psychologist-and-an-israeli-humanitarian-organization-are-helping-sierra-leone-stand-up-to-ebola-interview/.
Forman, A. (2014, October). Five words that can change the world. *Jewish Journal.* Retrieved from http://boston.forward.com/articles/185615/five-words-that-can-change-the-world/.
Hays, R. E., & Lyons, S. J. (1981). The bridge drawing: A projective technique for assessment in art therapy. *Arts in Psychotherapy, 8* , 207–17. doi: 10.1016/0197-4556(81) 90033-2.
International Child Art Foundation. (n.d.). Retrieved from www.icaf.org.
Jean-Charles, W. (2011a). *First international conference on restoring life and maintaining hope in Port-au-Prince: Establishing a new "Center for Spirituality and Mental Health" in Haiti, 15*(4), 39–41. Retrieved from http://internationalpsychology.files.wordpress.com/2013/01/ipbfall2011-10-28-1final.pdf.
Jean-Charles, W. (2011b, January–March). Rebati: After the earthquake, the IAAP UN team continues to remember Haiti. *IAAP Bulletin of the International Association of Applied Psychology, 23*(1/2), 33–35. Retrieved from http://www.new.iaapsy.org/uploads/newsletters/April2011.pdf.
Kuriansky, J. (2008). A clinical toolbox for cross-cultural counseling and training. In U. P. Gielen, J. G. Draguns, & J. M. Fish (eds), *Principles of multicultural counseling and therapy* (pp. 295–330). New York: Taylor and Francis/Routledge.
Kuriansky, J. (2010a, Spring). Haiti pre- and post-earthquake: Tracing professional and personal commitments, past, present, and future. *International Psychology Bulletin, 14*(2), 29–37. Retrieved from http://internationalpsychology.files.wordpress.com/2013/01/ipb_spring_2010_4_27_10.pdf.
Kuriansky, J. (2010b). Stories of Haiti. Retrieved from http://www.humnews.com/humnews/2010/4/13/stories-of-haitiapril-13-2010.html.
Kuriansky, J. (2011a). Aftermath of the Japanese earthquake and tsunami: Immediate response and impacts of events as healing efforts. *International Psychology Bulletin, 15*(2), 67–70. Retrieved from https://internationalpsychology.files.wordpress.com/2013/01/ipb_spring_2011-04-16-1-forrv-9-28-2011.pdf.
Kuriansky, J. (2011b, January–April.). Guidelines for mental health and psychosocial support in response to emergencies: Experience and encouragement for advocacy. *IAAP Bulletin. International Association of Applied Psychology Covering the World of Applied Psychology, 23*(1/2), 30–32. Retrieved from http://www.iaapsy.org/Portals/1/Bulletin/apnl_v23_i1-2.pdf.
Kuriansky, J. (2012a). Our communities: Healing after environmental disasters. In D. G. Nemeth, R. B. Hamilton, & J. Kuriansky (eds.), *Living in an environmentally traumatized world: Healing ourselves and our planet* (pp. 141–67). Santa Barbara, CA: Praeger.
Kuriansky, J. (2012b, July–October). Recovery efforts for Japan after the 3/11 devastating tsunami/earthquake. *Bulletin of the International Association of Applied Psychology, 24*(2/3), Part 22.
Kuriansky, J. (2012c). Report: Soothing Sendai. Retrieved from http://www.humnews.com/the-view-from-here/2012/3/22/soothing-sendai-report.html.
Kuriansky, J. (2013a, May). Helping kids cope with the Oklahoma tornado and other traumas: Seven techniques. *Huffington Post.* Retrieved from http://www.huffingtonpost.com/judy-kuriansky-phd/helping-kids-cope-with-the-oklahoma-tornado_b_3322238.html.
Kuriansky, J. (2013b). Superstorm Sandy 2012: A psychologist first responder's personal account and lessons learned about the impact on emotions and ecology. *Ecopsychology, 5*(S1), S-30–S-37. doi: 10.1089/eco.2013.0010. Retrieved from http://online.liebertpub.com/doi/abs/10.1089/eco.2013.0010?src=recsys.
Kuriansky, J. (2013c). Talking to kids about the anniversary of Superstorm Sandy. *Huffington Post.* Retrieved from https://www.huffpost.com/entry/talking-to-kids-about-the-anniversary-of-superstorm-sandy_n_4167294.
Kuriansky, J. (2013d). Thoughts on Katrina vs. Sandy: Essays on nature-induced, human-induced, and nature + human-induced environmental trauma. *Ecopsychology, 5*(S1), S-20-S-26. doi: 10.1089/eco.2013.0039. Retrieved from http://online.liebertpub.com/doi/abs/10.1089/eco.2013.0039?src=recsys .

Kuriansky, J. (2015). The role of community in the intersection of psychology and environmental protection. In D. G. Nemeth & J. Kuriansky (eds.), *Ecopsychology: Advances in the intersection of psychology and environmental protection, vol. 11: Interventions and policy* (pp. 419–24). Santa Barbara, CA: ABC-CLIO/Praeger.

Kuriansky, J. (2016a). Psychosocial support for a burial team: Gender issues and help for young men helping their country. In J. Kuriansky (ed.), *The psychosocial aspects of a deadly epidemic: What Ebola has taught us about holistic healing* (pp. 233–42). Santa Barbara, CA: ABC-CLIO/Praeger.

Kuriansky, J. (2016b, January). Report of the IAAP United Nations Team: Success in the New Global Agenda advocacy. *Bulletin of the International Association of Applied Psychology,* 28(1), 80–88.

Kuriansky, J. (ed.). (2016c). *The psychosocial aspects of a deadly epidemic: What Ebola has taught us about holistic healing.* Santa Barbara, CA: ABC-CLIO/Praeger.

Kuriansky, J. (2017). Réconstruire la raison et l'esprit en Haïti: Contributions du Centre de Spiritualité et de Santé Mentale [Rebuilding mind and spirit in Haiti: Accomplishments and gratifications of partnership with Father Wismick and CESSA]. In W. Jean-Charles (ed.), *Santé mentale et Psychothérapie en Haïti, Approches Intégratives et Traitements Multimodeaux* (pp. 1–15). Coconut Creek, FL: EducaVision. Retrieved from https://www.dropbox.com/personal?preview=Haiti+chapter+for+CESSA+book+Dr+Judy+Kuriansky+2017+May+20+FINAL+THIS+ONE+English.pdf.

Kuriansky, J. (2018, April). Psychotherapy, psychology, psychiatry, and international policy: Professional contributions and personal experiences about mental health and well-being, psychosocial resilience, and peace. *International Journal of Psychotherapy, Counseling, and Psychiatry: Theory, Research, and Clinical Practice. Special Volume of the World Council for Psychotherapy Conference 2017.* Retrieved from http://ijpcp.com/journal03/j30a06.pdf.

Kuriansky, J., & Jean-Charles, W. (2012, July–October). Haiti Rebati: Update on activities rebuilding Haiti through the Global Kids Connect Project. *Bulletin of the International Association of Applied Psychology, 24*(2/3), Part 21, 116–24.

Kuriansky, J., & Nemeth, D. G. (2013, September). A model for Post-Environmental Disaster Wellness Workshops: Preparing individuals and communities for hurricane anniversary reactions. *Ecopsychology, 5*(S1), S-38–S-45. doi: 10.1089/eco.2013.0006. Retrieved from http://online.liebertpub.com/doi/abs/10.1089/eco.2013.0006?src=recsys.

Kuriansky, J., Margevich, A., Jean-Charles, W., & Daisey, R. (2017). Resilience and recovery in natural disasters and epidemics: Comparisons, challenges, and lessons learned from Train-the-Trainer projects. In G. Rich & S. Sirikantraporn (eds.), *Human strengths and resilience: Developmental, cross-cultural, and international perspectives.* Lanham, MD: Lexington. Retrieved from https://www.amazon.com/Human-Strengths-Resilience-Developmental-Cross-Cultural/dp/1498554830/ref=mt_hardcover?_encoding=UTF8&me=.

Kuriansky, J., Polizer, Y., & Zinsou, J. (2016). Children and Ebola: A model Resilience and Empowerment Training and Workshop. In J. Kuriansky (Ed.), *The psychosocial aspects of a deadly epidemic: What Ebola has taught us about holistic healing* (pp. 175–214). Santa Barbara, CA: ABC-CLIO/Praeger.

Kuriansky, J., Wu, L-Y., Bao, C., Chand, D., Kong, S., Spooner, N., & Mao, S. (2015). Interventions by international and national organizations for psychosocial support after the Sichuan Earthquake in China: A review and implications for sustainable development. In D. G. Nemeth, J. Kuriansky, & R. Hamilton (eds.), *Ecopsychology: Advances in the intersection of psychology and environmental protection, vol. 11: Interventions and policy* (pp. 171–231). Santa Barbara, CA: ABC-CLIO/Praeger.

Kuriansky, J., Zinsou, J., Arunagiri, V., Douyon, C., Chiu, A., Jean-Charles, W., Daisey, R. & Midy, T. (2015). Effects of helping in a Train-the-Trainers program for youth in the Global Kids Connect Project after the 2010 Haiti earthquake: A paradigm shift to sustainable development. In D. G. Nemeth, J. Kuriansky, & R. Hamilton (eds.), *Ecopsychology: Advances in the intersection of psychology and environmental protection, vol. 11: Interventions and policy* (pp. 135–69). Santa Barbara, CA: ABC-CLIO/Praeger.

La Greca, A., Silverman, W., Vernberg, E. M., & Roberts, M. C. (eds.) (2002). *Helping children cope with disasters and terrorism*. Washington, DC: American Psychological Association.

Laor, N., Wolmer, L., Kora, M., Yucel, D., Spirman, S., & Yazgan, Y. (2002). Posttraumatic, dissociative, and grief symptoms in Turkish children exposed to the 1999 earthquakes. *Journal of Nervous and Mental Disease*, *190*, 824–32. doi: 10.1097/00005053-200212000-00004.

Malchiodi, C. (2005). Using art activities to support trauma recovery in children. *Trauma and Loss: Research and Interventions*, *5*(1), 8–11.

Masangkay, M. (2015). Psychologist connects disaster-affected children around the world. *Japan Times*. Retrieved from http://www.japantimes.co.jp/news/2015/03/23/national/psychologist-connects-disaster-affected-children-around-the-world/.

Nemeth, D. G. (2018). Starting over after environmental trauma. *International Journal of Psychotherapy, Counseling, and Psychiatry: Theory, Research, and Clinical Practice*, *3*, 1–9. Retrieved from http://ijpcp.com/journal03/j03a10.pdf.

Nemeth, D. G., & Olivier, T. (2017). *Innovative approaches to individual and community resilience: From theory to practice*. Amsterdam, The Netherlands: Elsevier.

Nemeth, D. G., Kuriansky, J., Olivier, T. W., Whittington, L. T., May, N., Hamilton, J., & Steger, A. (2011). Group interventions for disaster/trauma anniversary reactions. *Global Horizons: The Center for Policy and Resilience*, *4*(1), 51–64.

Nemeth, D. G., Kuriansky, J., Reeder, K. P., Lewis, A., Marceaux, K., Whittington, T., Olivier, T., May, N. E., & Safier, J. A. (2012). Addressing anniversary reactions of trauma through group process: The Hurricane Katrina Anniversary Wellness Workshops. *International Journal of Group Psychotherapy*, *62*(1), 129–41.

Osofsky, J. D. (ed.). (2004). *Young children and trauma: Intervention and treatment*. New York: Guilford Press.

Peveto, K. (2016, October). Workshops planned to help flood survivors become more resilient. *Advocate*. Retrieved from https://www.theadvocate.com/baton_rouge/entertainment_life/health_fitness/article_9973c6b8-9ba4-11e6-8a9e-e33e3bf8e108.html.

Rodin, J. (2014). *Being strong in a world where things go wrong: The resilience dividend*. New York: Public Affairs Publishing.

Smilan, C. (2009). Building resiliency to childhood trauma through arts-based learning. *Childhood Education*, *85*(6), 380–84.

UNISDR. (2015). The Sendai Framework for Disaster Risk Reduction 2015–2030. Retrieved from https://www.preventionweb.net/files/43291sendaiframework fordrren.pdf.

United Nations. (2015). The United Nations 2030 Agenda for Sustainable Development. Retrieved from https://sustainabledevelopment.un.org/content/documents/21252030%20Agenda%20for%20Sustainable%20Development%20web.pdfations.

Webb, N. (ed.). (2004). *Mass trauma and violence: Helping families and children cope*. New York: Guilford Press.

Yedida, T., & Itzahaky, H. (2004). A drawing technique for diagnosis and therapy of adolescents suffering traumatic stress and loss related to terrorism. In N. Webb (ed.), *Mass trauma and violence: Helping families and children cope* (pp. 283–303). New York: Guilford Press.

Zimmerman M. A. (2000). Empowerment theory. In J. Rappaport & E. Seidman (eds.), *Handbook of community psychology* (pp. 43–63). Boston: Springer.

Chapter Five

Dance Movement Therapy for Social Change

Working with Syrian and Rohingya Asylum Seekers

Seda S. Güney and Danny S. Lundmark

This chapter focuses on dance movement therapy (DMT) as a powerful tool for psychosocial support when working with asylum seekers (a term that will be used interchangeably with the term *refugees*), who have migrated due to war, conflict, or a general threat to their safety. The scope of this chapter focuses on work with two different populations through two different projects; the first one was with Syrian refugee children in Turkey, while the second addressed the needs of Rohingya women and girls in Bangladesh. Both projects focused on an integrated, trauma-informed, psychosocial support model, using multiple disciplines to address the needs of the populations. DMT techniques were used in collaboration with music therapy, art therapy, and photography or visual storytelling to provide care for the refugee populations and training for those who work with them.

One project started in 2014, designed as a five-day intensive program for a maximum of 60 Syrian refugee children between the ages of six and 12 years of age; it was subsequently repeated regularly with a different group of children (Güney, Atik, & Lundmark, 2018). These children, who had fled from war in Syria, had migrated to Istanbul, Turkey. The project was initiated in Istanbul, incorporating a team of arts therapists, volunteers, translators, and support staff.

The other project took place in 2018, in Cox's Bazaar, Bangladesh. It involved Rohingya asylum seekers who had fled from Myanmar (Burma) to Bangladesh, due to military operations launched by the Myanmar government (Hossain, Sultana, & Das, 2018). The participants had experienced mass murder, rape, torture, and displacement (Médecins sans Frontières, 2018). The project facilitators first worked with 45 local staff members, training them in psychosocial support methods; then they continued to work with two groups of Rohingya women and girls (totaling 46 participants) in the Kutupalong refugee camp, for five days, alongside 20 members of the local staff who had been in the training program.

In relation to the whole-person approach, both projects took into account the various needs and circumstances of the participants, with the project facilitators working together to adjust the programs when necessary. While many of the participants revealed symptoms of PTSD, they were not identified by their diagnosis; indeed, they were viewed as whole persons, with their family background, personal history, motivations, hopes, and dreams taken into account. This approach allowed for a wider perspective and accommodation of the personal needs of each participant. Although both projects were limited to a short-term time frame, the interventions and their results can be used to further the work of social workers, therapists, teachers, humanitarian aid workers, and psychosocial support workers who work with refugees.

DANCE MOVEMENT THERAPY AND THE WHOLE-PERSON APPROACH TO TRAUMA

Dance movement therapy is defined as the "use of movement to promote emotional, social, cognitive, and physical integration" (American Dance Therapy Association, 2016). As such, the definition largely applies to the whole-person approach, allowing therapists to relate to clients from a wider perspective. Harris (2007) notes that dance movement therapy helps clients to overcome cultural differences, while assisting participants in grounding themselves in their bodies. He also mentions that DMT is a flexible medium that can be applied to a variety of populations (p. 154).

The application of DMT to refugee populations who have experienced displacement and, oftentimes, physical and emotional violence offers an adaptable, nonlinguistic, and safe avenue of therapeutic intervention. According to Callaghan (1998), a number of factors make dance movement therapy a viable therapeutic medium for refugees. She explains that refugees often exhibit signs of decreased self-esteem, feelings of physical detachment, and psychosomatic symptoms, as well as difficulty using language to express and manage their emotions, including the use of words to protect themselves against emotions. These descriptions resemble the symptoms of PTSD.

PTSD is a diagnosis affecting the whole being of a person, resulting from either a single traumatizing event or from prolonged trauma(s). Typical symptoms of PTSD include "intrusive thoughts," "avoiding reminders," "negative thoughts and feelings," and "arousal and reactive symptoms" during a range of months or years (Parekh, 2017). Examples of these symptoms can be withdrawal and dissociation from surroundings, frequent flashbacks about the traumatizing event(s), nightmares and difficulty sleeping, feelings of isolation and/or loneliness, and behavioral problems. PTSD is a difficult diagnosis that cannot simply be cured through medication; it is a complex condition that usually requires long-term treatment, with the quality of life often negatively affected.

Rationale

DMT typically includes elements from trauma-informed practices, as its use of structured and improvised dance elements allows space for group creation and verbal reflection. Rothschild (2000) states that when approaching trauma, "psychological, neurobiological, and psychobiological" theories are helpful (p. xii), as trauma has a wide effect on the body and its systems. Therapists working with trauma should integrate verbal and movement therapy, while showing flexibility and adapting to the trauma(s) of their clients. Serlin (2007) writes that the

> major principles to consider when working with trauma through dance therapy include nonverbal mirroring and attunement, containment, developmental sequencing and reexperiencing, and working through of bodily held blocks and issues. Because dance/movement therapy is action-oriented and spontaneous, it is creative and works with mind, body, and spirit. (p. 113)

In DMT sessions, group warm-ups and body awareness exercises often are used to prepare the group to reduce the risk of body injuries, while building a connection among the group members. In the two projects described in this chapter, working with groups demonstrated social interaction and collaboration with others, while giving importance to personal space and boundaries. Understanding the use of body weight and props in relation to others helped to address both the physical and social aspects of moving within the group.

According to Levine, Land, and Lizano (2015), dance therapists working with women with PTSD have mentioned numerous common elements in their approaches. Some of these are warm-up, movement, metaphor, body awareness, mirroring, empowerment, trust, self-care, and integration of other modalities. DMT as an integrative care model can be a tool for assessing needs, building trust and communication skills, creating a sense of safety, encouraging freedom of expression, and developing healthy boundaries.

Dancing in the space as a group brought a sense of togetherness, as the community integrated drama exercises, gestures, and voice to create a safe space to express and manage difficult emotions, with the support of the group. These exercises supported individuals physically, socially, spiritually, emotionally, and psychologically. The freedom of choice, initiation, participation, and building of connections were reinforced through the other modalities.

CREATING A SAFE SPACE

It is important that any therapeutic work take place in a space that is safe and conducive to the freedom of expression. This is especially significant for populations who have experienced war, which usually involves torture, rape, and mass displacement. The effects of these extreme circumstances can leave individuals feeling lost and hopeless. As Meyer (1999) writes, "Under torture and violence, the boundaries of the 'house of the body' are invaded. To protect itself, the individual will lock the doors, close the window, turn off the lights, and hide in the dark" (p. 242). It was important for participants in these projects to feel safe both in their bodies and within the setting. Dieterich-Hartwell and Koch (2017) specifically suggest that creative arts therapies be used to create a temporary home.

Creating a safe space on both a physical and an interconnected (social) level was crucial for therapeutic work to occur. This safe space needed to be built with the active involvement of the community, the therapist, volunteers, and participants to serve the needs of everyone. According to research in the field, interventions should promote a safe and calm atmosphere, fostering feelings of both individual and communal efficiency, hope, and connectedness (Betancourt et al., 2013; Shibley & Stoddard, 2011; Barenbaum, Ruchkin, & Shwab-Stone, 2004; Attanayake et al., 2009; Inter-Agency Standing Committee, 2007; United Nations Children's Fund, 2011; Shaw, Espinel, & Shultz, 2012; Stoddard & Saxe, 2001).

PHYSICAL SAFE SPACE

The physical space in which the sessions took place was significant, so it was considered with great care. As the result of creating a safe environment and maximizing the efficiency of space, sessions were organized to run smoothly, ensuring the best practice possible from team members and participants. Past physical spaces have been tents, classrooms, outdoor areas, or other areas designated by the aid organization.

For the participants to move more comfortably, doors, floors, windows, lighting, and the temperature of the atmosphere were checked to minimize any risks while moving. For example, circles were marked or chairs were set up and organized in the space to help participants focus and feel safe from the moment when they arrived. This was to help them cope with the anxiety

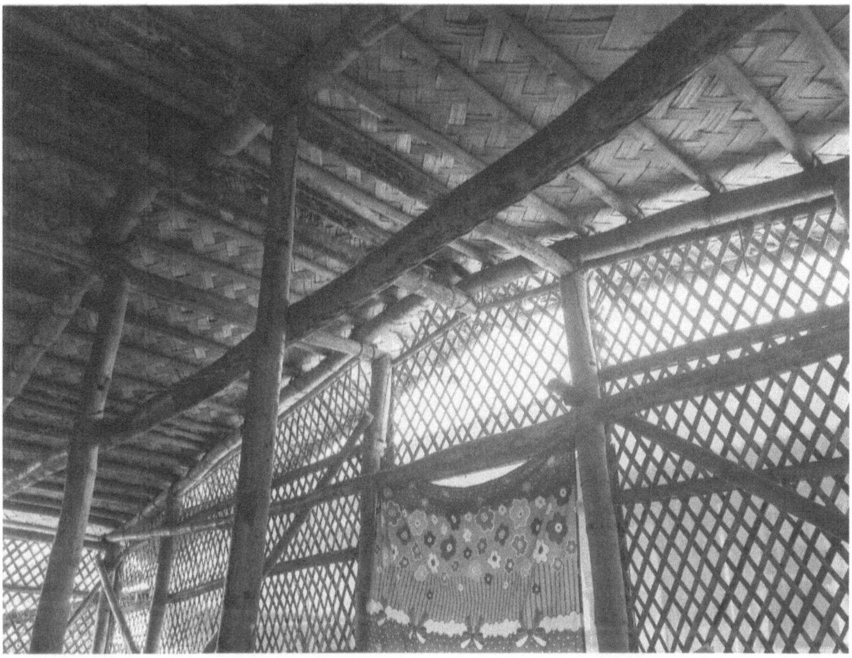

Figure 5.1. The therapy space at the camp. *Danny S. Lundmark*

of entering a new space, enabling them to have a better understanding of where they were to sit or stand. This space, which changed according to the needs of the groups, required rearrangement between sessions.

In addition, there was a culturally sensitive element to the organization of physical space, as, for example, members of some cultures felt more comfortable sitting on the floor as opposed to chairs. In Bangladesh, the space was covered with colorful materials for both privacy and decorative reasons. During the project, the space transformed creatively with drawings, photos, scarves, and additions by the participants and team members. Decoration of the space became a process, as the physical space was cocreated by the participants. Meyer (1999) speaks about a waiting room for asylum seekers and how, when she initiated sessions, the room was transformed into a "play room," allowing a creative space for group work. It became not only a physical space, but also a "play room" (p. 248).

INTERCONNECTED SPACE/BECOMING A GROUP

In addition to provision of a safe physical space, a connection between personal and group space was needed. Bar-Sinai (Serlin, Berger, & Bar-Sinai, 2007) mentions that both the personal space and the group space developed "responsibility, commitment, and dialogue in a pluralistic atmosphere" (pp. 373–74).

The verbal and nonverbal group agreements were a good example of an interconnected safe space where everyone in the group could feel both safe and heard. Such group agreements were essential, as they helped to create an atmosphere where participants could discover what was personally significant for each individual. The agreement was one of the first activities with the refugee groups and was considered to be one of the core requirements to create a safe, interconnected space. Building consensus on a set of agreements, the framing of boundaries, and needs helped the group to own the time shared together, allowing each participant to be heard clearly. The group agreement process presented opportunities for concerns, hopes, and expectations, helping the entire group to show more respect and allowing opportunities for individual participation.

Drawing on the therapeutic contract, it was important to discuss confidentiality, equality, respect for differences, and openness to new experiences. While the groups were developing their own agreements, there were certain points that the project team encouraged them to include as part of the contract. For example, it was important to include the idea of "listening," which would allow every member of the group to be heard. The age of participants greatly influenced how much the facilitators added to the group agreement, with younger participants needing more direction than adults. In addition, the agreement had to be flexible enough to give space to new additions, as the group process continued. For example, it was surprising when the Rohingya girls group added the word *dream* to the group agreement. This provided another level of cocreating to the agreement within the group, allowing for dreams and hopes for the future. Overall, the use of a group agreement helped participants and team members foster a mutually safer, more reliable, and more efficient therapeutic atmosphere.

Among the agreements, confidentiality was crucial, especially on behalf of the project team. The ideas of privacy and consent were an important aspect of creating a safe space, as they gave reassurance to the participants that their involvement and any content created would be confidential and limited within the confines of the workspace. For the Rohingya women and girls' groups, this was particularly important, as the workshops took place inside the refugee camps in Bangladesh.

There was also a difference between visibility and confidentiality. The therapeutic work tended to be limited to the space where the work was

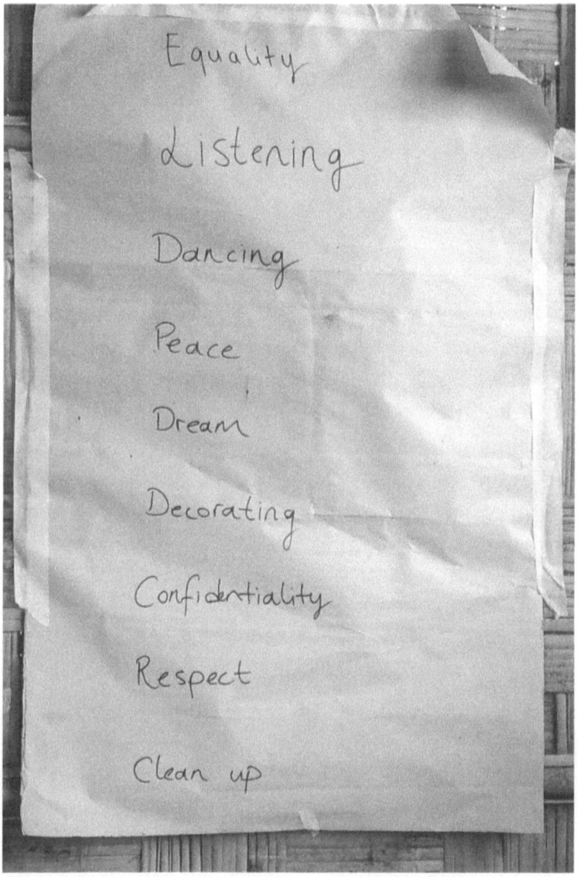

Figure 5.2. The group agreement. *Danny S. Lundmark*

conducted; however, it contributed to the community on social, spiritual, emotional, physical, and psychological levels as well. The visibility issue was discussed among the team members with one of their colleagues, who was a photographer and a visual storyteller. He emphasized the importance of the correspondence between empowerment and visibility. The facilitator team agreed that any shared content needed to be handled with care and attention, and with the full permission of anyone involved. Logistics, cultural sensitivities, and the general rules of the refugee camp, school, or setting needed to be taken into consideration when agreeing on elements of working together.

CARE FOR THE CAREGIVERS

While working with trauma, it was essential to provide psychosocial support workers and other staff members with skills related to self-care. This included information about trauma-sensitive techniques, prevention from burnout, and compassion fatigue. To support the beneficiaries, the facilitators first had to support their own team members, enabling them to support themselves as well. As each team member relied on the others, a solid foundation was established among them. The important aspect about training the team was that they had a chance to experience the modalities, thereby learning from first-person experience. In this way, they could apply the techniques safely, within their abilities and qualifications.

Every member of the team of translators, psychosocial support workers, and community mobilizers was involved in the decision-making process, which helped maintain flexibility, cultural sensitivity, and awareness. Feedback from the entire team was key. The nature of humanitarian aid and cultural sensitivities had to be understood and taken into account; any concerns or questions about techniques needed to be considered and integrated into the program accordingly. For example, in Bangladesh, there were both Bengali and Rohingya women in the same group, with the Bengali psychosocial support officers (who were involved in the training program) helping to support the Rohingya refugees.

Both of these cultures differed from the cultures of the therapists. Thus, there seemed to be power dynamics at work both within and across the communities. Thus, even though there seemed to be hierarchies within both the Rohingya and the Bengali communities, the facilitators stressed the importance of group agreement and equality; once in the group circle, each person was to be liberated from any hierarchical constraints, allowing each of them the opportunity to both follow and lead activities. This seemed to be difficult for those who closely identified with either the "leader" or the "follower" position in their ordinary day-to-day relations. Indeed, there were several times when participants' preconceived ideas about their own identity seemed to limit their interactions within the group.

The facilitators were keen to develop the cognitive, physical, and emotional skills of the beneficiaries, as well as those of the local staff. The beneficiaries also played an important role in the decision-making process, as the flexibility offered by the facilitators allowed for an adaptive approach that could integrate spontaneous needs and decisions. The participants were working through their own personal trauma(s) and need(s) in the groups, and, as Serlin, Berger, and Bar-Sinai (2007) note, the nonverbal action of dance could help provide resolution of conflict by providing a better understanding of cultural differences.

The therapists themselves were also influenced by cultural differences. Being abroad in an emergency setting was different from being in their hometowns, with the unfamiliarity of the environment requiring more than ever that the therapists be able to care for themselves both during and outside of sessions. In working with a population that had suffered extreme violence, the nature of the work was emotionally challenging. It was easy to appreciate the difficulties experienced by the participants, as well as their challenging living conditions. At the same time, it was essential that the facilitators care for themselves. As Meyer (1999) asks, "How can I, as a therapist, protect myself and stay at home in my body?" (p. 241).

Some of the tools that the therapists used to process their own thoughts and feelings included the use of professional and peer supervision; communication with friends and family; mindful meditation, journal writing, art, and/or music making; and other favorite rituals that could help release their emotions.

DANCE MOVEMENT THERAPY WITH DIVERSITY, ETHNICITY, AND GENDER

Among refugees, such topics as diversity, ethnicity, and gender played an important role during the course of therapeutic intervention. Participants in the groups came from a wide range of places, whether from within a single country or from several countries. There was a high probability of ethnic diversity, as well as geographic diversity, reflecting different religious, national, and cultural backgrounds. A similar diversity applied to gender and preconceived notions about gender roles within the population. As such, it was important for the facilitators in any project working with displaced people to approach their work with cultural sensitivity, as well as an open mind about what to expect from participants. With an inclusive and respectful approach, therapists and facilitators could learn about their clients to develop better and more culturally sensitive strategies for their work together.

When groups were working with the music therapist, the cultural diversity was readily apparent. A few of the Bengali psychosocial support staff spoke two different dialects of Bangla, including a Chittagonian dialect. Some of the Rohingya beneficiaries spoke the Chittagonian dialect, but they also spoke other dialects, and the use of translators was crucial for the group members to understand one another. To compound the situation, the facilitators spoke English, while not understanding any of the other dialects. Despite the apparent complexity of the situation, song lyrics were written using a mix of Rohingya, Bengali, and Indian dialects, in addition to a modicum of English. The mix of languages allowed for an inclusive and nondiscriminatory approach, and, with the use of live music, an extremely adaptable atmosphere was created, enabling the participation of every group member.

The use of music was also an important aspect within the DMT sessions. A wide variety of music needed to be available to match the needs and energy levels of the groups. When live music was involved, the music therapist carefully improvised with the group, while maintaining awareness of group dynamics and movements, thus helping to support the needs of the group. In the case of recorded music, the groups were often consulted, and culturally appropriate music was played according to suggestions made by the participants.

It was interesting to observe how music influenced the dance. Movements seemed to be more authentic when the music therapist improvised and became more stylized when a cultural song was played (e.g., Indian music). A great deal of emotional releasing was observed in the celebratory dances during the last days with both the Syrian and Rohingya refugees; moreover, the photographs and artworks also changed and were more expressive. In the case of the Syrian refugees, music therapy sessions happened simultaneously in a different room, while the dance movement therapist regularly used recorded music. During the project with the Rohingya refugees, however, the music therapist was in the same space, coleading with the dance movement therapist and supporting the movement process.

It was moving to see the Rohingya women and girls integrating a wide mixture of dances into their work. Participants used a variety of Indian dances, for instance, the Bharatanatyam, Bengali dances, and other traditional Eastern movements, as well as religious rituals and commercialized Eastern and Western dances. Later in the process, improvised dance, expressive movement, and rhythmic coherence were observed. The participants' use of props enabled a playful environment for both projects. Feelings of shyness, reluctance, and immobility often gave way to a playful, relaxed, and fun atmosphere, as participants danced together to assorted rhythms.

Overall, the coordination among music therapy, art therapy, visual storytelling, and dance movement therapy was creative and complementary, forming a therapeutic support process as a "multilayered process of holding together" (Butte & Whelan, 2018, p. 57).

EVALUATION

To understand the efficacy of the programs, evaluations were made at the end of both projects. A study conducted regarding the project with Syrian refugee children found that depression, trauma, and trait anxiety symptoms were significantly reduced afterward. This was determined by a pre- and postassessment using the Stressful Life Events questionnaire, the UCLA Posttraumatic Stress Disorder Parent Version, and the Child Depression Inventory (Ugurlu, Akca, & Acarturk, 2016).

For the Rohingya project, a qualitative, participatory evaluation method called the "Most Significant Change" (Davies & Dart, 2005) was adapted, with not only the Rohingya women and girls, but also the Bengali psychosocial support workers. This process of receiving feedback from the members acted as an assessment for the effectiveness of the project. They were asked about the most significant change that had taken place in their lives since the project began, why this change was significant, would this project change any actions/thoughts/behaviors in the future, and was there anything additional they would like to share. Hearing about the most significant changes from first-person narratives was very powerful. Many of the participants had become active agents in determining the changes and assessing their own needs for further development.

One of the most significant changes that took place was empowerment of the participants. Many refugees reported feeling more confident, safe, and happy. The project helped them to relieve stress, as well as learn new skills. There also were numerous reflections from participants. Many stated that they felt less shy than before the project, as they had learned to take the initiative and exercised leadership skills. This was notable, as many beneficiaries noted that they never had these opportunities before the program. Support workers also shared their most significant changes, with their reflections showing that they also had been very engaged in the process and empowered to apply the skills to meet their own needs, as well as the needs of the community. After the project was completed, the Bengali psychosocial support workers, with input from the Rohingya participants, created their own curriculum using creative arts, movement, music, and photography. This was a promising development, as the tools and concepts provided by the initial project were thereby sustained long after the project's completion.

QUALIFICATION AND TRAINING REQUIREMENTS

To work as a dance movement psychotherapist, one must train in a dance movement psychotherapy course at a master's level with an accredited organization or university. This requirement may differ, of course, according to country regulations. At the same time, professional registration with a relevant dance movement psychotherapy association is essential for the establishment of a safe practice. An open attitude toward learning is recommended, as well as experience working within the community. Attendance at continuous professional development trainings in the field of trauma-informed practices and supervision is also useful. It is important to work with a team, for example, workshop facilitators, therapists, and social workers.

The work mentioned in this chapter has impacted Syrian refugee children in Istanbul, Turkey, as well as Rohingya women and girls in the gender-based violence (GBV) unit in Cox's Bazaar, Bangladesh. NGO facilitators, teachers, translators, dancers, photographers, community mobilizers, psychosocial support workers, social workers, arts therapists, psychologists, pedagogues, and activists have participated in these projects. This teamwork supports not only the war-affected populations, but also those who work with these populations.

DISCUSSION AND CONCLUSION

Overall, the use of DMT, as an integrated model, when working with refugees, along with the myriad creative collaborations, supported the participants in finding their own strength and resources. By performing a solo dance, the participants noticed and appreciated their unique abilities, leading to an increase in their self-esteem. Being mirrored by the group helped them to be seen and heard, expressing their needs and trusting in themselves more. Experiencing leadership activities helped them to make decisions in the moment, also prompting their imaginations. The act of forming dances together was a creative and healing process of coexisting with others in the group, while shared rhythms and movements supported transformation and growth. Shared dance performances not only nourished the participants, but also encouraged them to develop their creative and artistic skills.

ACKNOWLEDGMENTS

We would like to acknowledge our dear colleagues: Leyla Akca Atik, Emir and Esra Özsüer, the Maya Foundation, Elco van der Wilt and Society Fresh, Tasha Colbert, Megan Denise Smith, and the International Organization for Migration-Bangladesh.

REFERENCES

American Dance Therapy Association (2016). What is dance/movement therapy? Retrieved from https://adta.org/faqs/.

Attanayake, V., McKay, R., Joffres, M., Singh, S., Burkle, F., & Mills, E. (2009). Prevalence of mental disorders among children exposed to war: A systematic review of 7,920 children. *Medicine Conflict and Survival, 25*(1), 4–19.

Barenbaum, J., Ruchkin, V., & Schwab-Stone, M. (2004). The psychological aspects of children exposed to war: Practice and policy initiatives. *Journal of Child Psychology and Psychiatry, 45*(1), 41–62.

Betancourt, T. S., Meyers-Ohki, S. E., Charrow, A. P., & Tol, W. A. (2013, March/April). Interventions for children affected by war: An ecological perspective on psychosocial support and mental health care. *Harvard Review of Psychiatry, 21*(2), 70–91.

Butte, C., & Whelan, D. (2018). Ambivalence, boundaries, edges, and expansion: Relatedness and collaboration in a dance movement psychotherapy and music therapy group for adults with learning disabilities. In T. Colbert & C. Bent (eds.), *Working across modalities in the arts therapies: Creative collaborations* (pp. 55–68). New York: Routledge.

Callaghan, K. (1998). In limbo: Movement psychotherapy with refugees and asylum seekers. In D. Dokter (ed.), *Art therapists, refugees and migrants: Reaching across borders* (pp. 25–40). London: Jessica Kingsley.

Davies, R., & Dart, J. (2005). The "most significant change" (MSC) technique: A guide to its use. Retrieved from http://www.mande.co.uk/wp-content/uploads/2005/MSCGuide.pdf.

Dieterich-Hartwell, R., & Koch, S. C. (2017). Creative arts therapies as temporary home for refugees: Insights from literature and practice. *Behavioral Sciences*, *7*(4), 69.

Güney, S. S., Atik, L. A., & Lundmark, D. S. (2018). Holding hope: Rehabilitation of Syrian refugee children through art, music, and dance movement therapy. In T. Colbert & C. Bent (eds.), *Working across modalities in the arts therapies: Creative collaborations* (pp. 95–108). New York: Routledge.

Harris, D. A. (2007). Dance/movement therapy approaches to fostering resilience and recovery among African adolescent torture survivors. *Torture*, *17*(2), 134–55.

Hossain, M. M., Sultana, A., & Das, A. (2018). Gender-based violence among Rohingya refugees in Bangladesh: A public health challenge. *Indian Journal of Medical Ethics*, *3*(3), 260. Retrieved from http://ijme.in/wp-content/uploads/2018/06/263le260genderbased.pdf.

Inter-Agency Standing Committee. (2007). *IASC guidelines on mental health and psychosocial support in emergency settings*. Geneva, Switzerland: IASC.

Levine, B., Land, H. M., & Lizano, E. L. (2015). The elements of dance/movement therapy employed when treating women with posttraumatic stress disorder. *Critical Social Work*, *16*(1), 40–57.

Médecins sans Frontières. (2018). "No one was left": Death and violence against the Rohingya in Rakhine state, Myanmar. Retrieved from https://www.doctorswithoutborders.ca/article/no-one-was-left-msf-special-report-violence-against-rohingya-myanmars-rakhine-state.

Meyer, M. A. (1999). In exile from the body: Creating a "play room" in the "waiting room." In E. G. Levine & S. K. Levine (eds.), *Foundations of expressive arts therapy: Theoretical and clinical perspectives* (pp. 241–55). Philadelphia, PA: Jessica Kingsley.

Parekh, R. (2017). What is posttraumatic stress disorder? *American Psychiatric Association*. Retrieved from https://www.psychiatry.org/patients-families/ptsd/what-is-ptsd.

Rothschild, B. (2000). *The body remembers: The psychophysiology of trauma and trauma treatment*. New York: W. W. Norton.

Serlin, I. A. (2007). Theory and practices of arts therapies: Whole-person integrative approaches to healthcare. In I. A. Serlin, J. Sonke-Henderson, R. Brandman, & J. Graham-Pole (eds.), *Whole-person healthcare: Vol. 3: The arts and health* (pp. 107–19). San Francisco, CA: Union Street Health Associates Press.

Serlin, I. A., Berger, M. R., & Bar-Sinai, R. (2007). Moving through conflict: Understanding personal and cultural differences through movement style. *Journal of Humanistic Psychology*, *47*(3), 367–75.

Shaw, J. A., Espinel, Z., & Shultz, J. M. (2012). *Care of children exposed to the traumatic effects of disaster*. Arlington, VA: American Psychiatric Publishing.

Shibley, H. L., & Stoddard, F. J., Jr. (2011). Child and adolescent psychiatry interventions. In F. J. Stoddard Jr., A. Pandya, & C. L. Katz (eds.), *Disaster psychiatry: Readiness, evaluation, and treatment* (pp. 287–312). Arlington, VA: American Psychiatric Publishing.

Stoddard, F. J., & Saxe, G. (2001). Ten-year research review of physical injuries. *Journal of the American Academy of Child and Adolescent Psychiatry*, *40*(10), 1,128–45.

Ugurlu, N., Akca, L., & Acarturk, C. (2016). An art therapy intervention for symptoms of posttraumatic stress, depression, and anxiety among Syrian refugee children. *Vulnerable Children and Youth Studies*, *11*(2), 89–102.

United Nations Children's Fund. (2011). *The state of the world's children: Adolescence, an age of opportunity*. New York: UNICEF.

Chapter Six

Animal-Assisted Interventions with Those Who Are Traumatized

Suzanne R. Engelman

This chapter focuses on the integrative and complementary healing approach of animal-assisted interventions (AAI) with those who are traumatized. Since conventional treatment methods of trauma-focused psychotherapy and/or medications often are not effective, an alternative modality called AAI is presented. Centered on the whole-person approach to health, the often-overlooked spiritual dimension as experienced through AAI is elucidated through the important human–animal bond.

THE WHOLE-PERSON APPROACH AND AAI

Trauma creates emotional constriction and disconnection, both within the traumatized individual and between that person and others. AAI is effective in integrating bio-psycho-social-spiritual aspects of well-being for the traumatized person through a spiritual model of change. The meaning of *spiritual* in this context consists of the elements of "experiencing wholeness and interconnectedness" (Kabat-Zinn, 1994, p. 266) and "love, kindness, and affection" (Dalai Lama, 2011, p. 17).

This spiritual model of AAI emphasizes the healing of the withdrawal and suffering that result from trauma through three processes: 1) the transpersonal proclivity to attach to animals; 2) the psychophysiological level of love and the bonding neurochemistry of oxytocin between humans and animals; and 3) a posttraumatic growth (PTG) expansion into interacting more meaningfully with others, "with changed priorities and a richer existential and spiritual life" (Tedeschi & Calhoun, 2004, p. 1). For example,

> The neurobiology of "we" is the sense that we can promote the integration of two or more individual systems into a larger functional whole. This sense of a "we" is at the heart of "feeling felt" that may be the simplest way of describing love. It is perhaps this deep sense of interpersonal integration that is also the heart of healing. (Siegel, 2010, p. 245)

Simply stated, for the traumatized person, this neurobiology of interrelatedness begins again with an animal, as it eases suffering within the person and then extends to relationships with other human beings.

CONVENTIONAL MODELS OF TRAUMA TREATMENT

Research indicates that, when using conventional treatment methods, a "majority of traumatized service members and veterans" go without sufficient remediation (Lefkowitz et al., 2005, p. 277). Others fail even to engage in treatment when it is offered to them (Hundt et al., 2017).

The reasons for ineffective or no treatment are manifold. They include fear of stigmatization; difficulty tolerating the discomfort of the traumatic reactions being retriggered; or avoidance of therapists, as interpersonally inflicted traumas may be complex and result in a "persistent distrust of others" (Tedeschi et al., 2015, p. 306), along with social withdrawal and isolation. Because psychotherapy is highly interpersonal in nature, attaining a therapeutic alliance in these cases may, therefore, fail. Such demographic factors as age, gender, race and ethnicity, social environment, and pretreatment symptoms also relate to this underuse or lack of effectiveness (Kehle-Forbes & Kimerling, 2017).

Since 1958, the VA has provided service dogs for veterans who have physical disabilities, for instance, limited mobility, vision, or hearing; unfortunately, the VA has not provided AAI services for its members who are traumatized or have other psychological disabilities (Weinmeyer, 2015). These problems further underscore the need for additional complementary treatment options like AAI, which may be more acceptable to those who are traumatized but do not use conventional methods or find them to be ineffective.

HISTORY OF AND GENETIC BOND TO ANIMALS

Throughout history, humankind has long valued its bond with animals. In mythology, the dog, in particular, is "commonly represented as an intermediary between this world and the next" (Eliade, 1964, p. 92). The respected relationship of animals to humans has been recorded in prehistoric hunting and foraging cultures that held animistic beliefs imbuing animals with supernatural powers. The continuing effects of animism and the power of animal spirits to guard humans' success and health are also seen in multiple early societies that employed shamanism (Eliade, 1964), where the shaman was empowered after entering a trance-like state by taking on the special healing powers of particular animals. "By becoming this mythical animal, man became something far greater and stronger than himself . . . and found a new dimension of life: spontaneity, freedom, 'sympathy' with all the cosmic rhythms, and, hence, bliss and immortality" (Eliade, 1964, p. 460). This is indicative of both a "hypersuggestible" (Grob, 1994, p. 7) state and the spiritual concept of PTG.

According to the evolutionary psychology hypothesis of biophilia, first proposed by Wilson (1984), humans have an "instinctive esthetic preference for natural environments and subconscious affiliation for other living organisms" (cited in Seymour, 2016, p. 2), as part of the species' search for meaning and a way to maintain health. Human neurophysiology may be preferentially "wired" to bond with animals due to its phylogenetic inheritance and as a deep way to reach inner emotions (Tedeschi et al., 2015). Other studies have shown that there are specialized neurons on the top of the amygdala in the human brain that respond only to animals (Knobloch-Bollmann et al., 2012). In addition, these neurons prefer to process pictures of animals rather than people or landmarks (Mormann et al., 2012).

WHAT IS AAI?

"AAI is a goal-oriented and structured intervention that intentionally includes or incorporates animals in health, education, and human services (e.g., social work), for the purpose of therapeutic gains in humans" (International Association of Human–Animal Interactions Organization [IAHAIO], 2014, p. 4). There are many varieties of AAI, differentiated by the type of animals used, their training, and the intentions of their role. The most commonly used animals in AAI are dogs; horses; and a smaller number of farm animals, like cats, sheep, pigs, chickens, opossums, and llamas (O'Haire, Guérin, & Kirkham, 2015), and parrots (Altschuler, 2018). The different types of AAI are briefly described here, followed by a discussion of how AAI may work to relieve suffering from the effects of trauma.

Canine Assistance-Interactions

These may include service dogs (SD), psychiatric service dogs (PSD), therapy dogs (TD), emotional support dogs (ESD), and companion dogs (CD). The settings for canine-assisted interactions are quite variable.

Service Dogs

Service dogs (SD) are working dogs that are extensively trained to respond precisely to specific disabilities of their owners, for example, blindness, deafness, paralysis, seizures, diabetes, and cardiac arrhythmias. They have legal protections under the American with Disabilities Act (ADA) regarding being in public places, as well as living in the owner's residence (U.S. Department of Justice, 2011).

Psychiatric Service Dogs

Psychiatric service dogs (PSD) have been trained to respond to psychiatric symptoms of their owners, including PTSD (Krause-Parello, Sarni, & Padden, 2016). Service dogs may be trained by their owners with additional professional guidance or be already trained to respond to the specific disability of the owner.

Therapy Dogs

Therapy dogs (TD), which are used in animal-assisted therapy (AAT), are selected for their agreeable dispositions, obedience-trained, and certified together with their owners by authorized examiners as a compatible therapy dog team. These dogs may frequent inpatient or outpatient facilities and are therapeutic for the people with whom they interact. AAT is a structured therapeutic intervention, with specific goals (Lundqvist et al., 2017), that enhances whatever activities its animals are involved in for people other than their owners.

Emotional Support Dogs

Emotional support dogs (ESD) have not been trained but are used to provide emotional comfort and companionship to their owners, who suffer from emotional distress or disabilities.

Companion Dogs

Companion dogs (CD), like ESDs, are untrained and largely considered to be their owners' pets.

Equine-Assisted Interactions (between a Human and a Horse)

Horses have played a historically important role in war. In other contexts, the power of horses and their instinctual desire to fit into a herd for safety make them positive AAI animals.

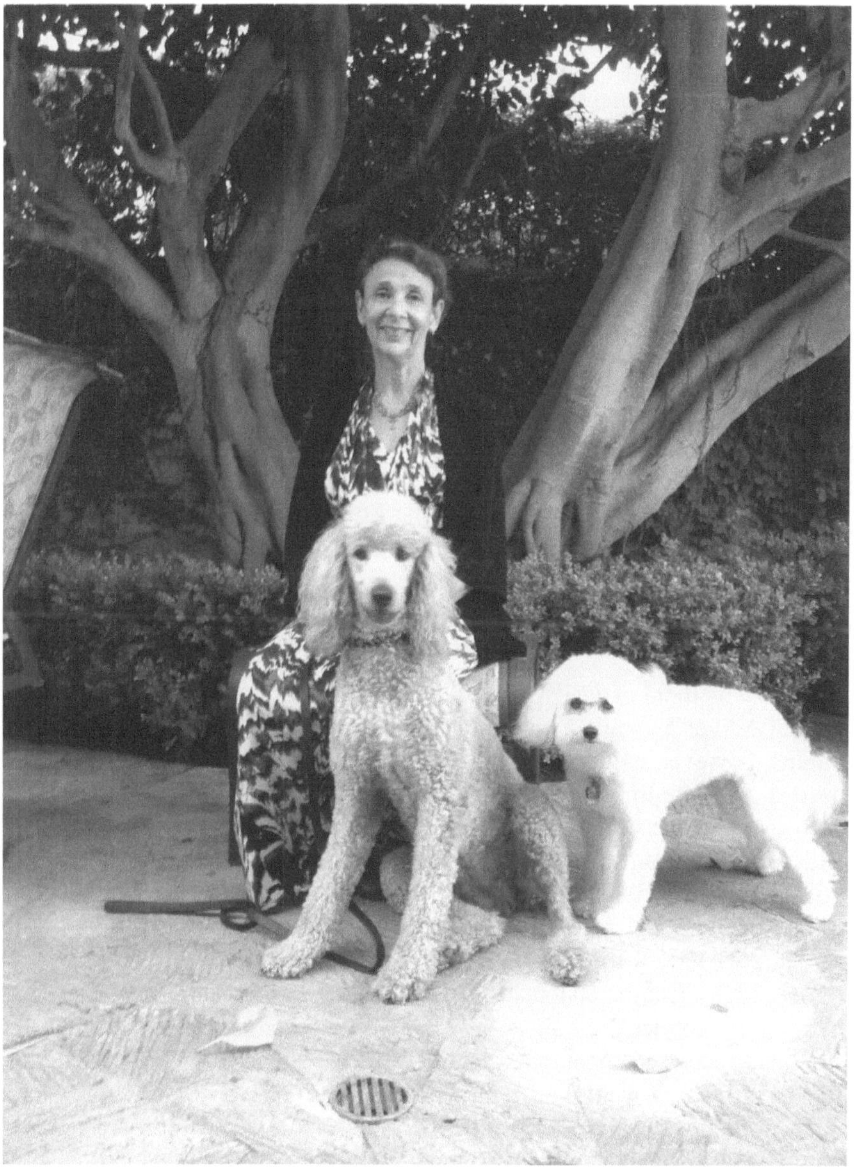

Figure 6.1. Dr. Engelman with her AAT cotherapists, Lizzy and CJ. ***Dennis E. O'Reilly***

Equine-Assisted Therapy and Equine-Assisted Counseling

Equine-assisted therapy (EAT) and equine-assisted counseling (EAC) both involve hippotherapy, or horseback riding, in which the horse's movements are used as the treatment intervention (Nevins et al., 2013).

Equine-Facilitated Psychotherapy

In equine-facilitated psychotherapy (EFP), the therapeutic intervention consists of becoming mindful of the thoughts and feelings that result from observing, grooming, and training a horse. Horses, which mirror human gestures and physiology, may provide immediate responses to a person's nonverbal behavior (e.g., horses may crowd a person who is hunched and avoiding eye contact or back away from a person who is approaching quickly with prolonged eye contact), "helping increase awareness of one's behaviors and emotions" (Earles, Vernon, & Yetz, 2015, p. 150).

The settings for equine-assisted interaction are mostly conducted in outdoor farms and riding centers. Bright Star Equestrian Center and the Saratoga WarHorse Connection program are two EAT facilities for veterans.

AAI EVIDENCE-BASED RESEARCH FOR PTSD

There is a plethora of anecdotal and qualitative studies showing the effectiveness of AAI as a complementary treatment modality for those suffering from trauma; however, evidence-based studies are limited, and additional ones are needed with control groups, larger sample sizes, and highly standardized protocols and measures. More empirical studies exist using canines but fewer with horses and other animals. Canines are the "only species used in traditional, clinic-based therapy sessions" (O'Haire, Guérin, & Kirkham, 2015, p. 5). Evidence-based research includes one recent proof of concept study showing AAI's effectiveness in reducing trauma symptoms (O'Haire & Rodriguez, 2018). Compared to usual care alone, "military members and veterans with trained service dogs show lower PTSD symptomology, reduced depression, and increased social participation" (p. 186). In 10 earlier AAI studies, PTSD symptoms were also reduced (O'Haire, Guérin, & Kirkham et al., 2015). Lundqvist et al. (2017) identified 14 randomized control studies presenting at least one significant positive effect in reducing psychiatric symptoms. Another review of 12 AAI studies showed positive effects with childhood trauma (Hoagwood et al., 2017). Nine AAI studies with horses showed reduction of PTSD symptoms (Staudt & Cherry, 2017). Finally, the VA is conducting a congressionally mandated study with people in the military to examine the impact of AAI on PTSD, intended to address the methodological weaknesses of prior studies (Saunders et al., 2017).

That said, it must also be noted that empirically validating efficacy when working in the realm of the spirit is far from easy. Indeed, "it will not be sufficient to adhere to strict standards of scientific methodology alone. We must also pay heed to the examples provided us by such successful applications of the shamanic paradigm," wherein "hypersuggestible properties" may be put to good use (Grob, 1994, p. 7). This paradigm emphasizes the importance of integrating the setting, meaning, and cultural and community norms, all of which affect the results of using AAI with trauma. Unlike usual evidence-based methods, the shamanic model respects that "hypersuggestibility" and healing can be enhanced by including these factors, as well as our historical interrelatedness to animals.

Transpersonal Explanations of AAI Effectiveness

Noted psychiatrist Carl Jung (1966) discussed animal symbols as being "transpersonal," or representing the "residues of functions from man's animal ancestry" (p. 98), deeply embedded in the human psyche, perhaps through archetypes rooted in what Jung referred to as the "collective unconscious." Similarly, Boris Levinson (1969) postulated that health is arrived at when a healthy connection is reestablished with one's inner, unconscious animal nature, by forming a helpful bond with present-day animals. Thus, the success of AAI may be the result of the traumatized person (through connection with an animal) coming to a "rewinding of the patient's unconscious to the very primitive phases of development . . . [the] temporally very ancient, and yet present, sane portion of his unconscious" (Carminati et al., 2013, p. 451). This phenomenon can then be generalized to human interactions, which, according to Stephen W. Porges (a Distinguished University Scientist at the Kinsey Institute), are the stuff of recovery: "We can't survive well without interacting with another appropriate mammal," be it dog or human (cited in National Institute for the Clinical Application of Behavioral Medicine, 2016, p. 23).

Perhaps a relationship with animals through what Jung conceptualized as the shared, deep, ancient, collective unconscious may allow for "partial reparation of dysfunctional upper layers" that include trauma symptoms (Carminati et al., 2013, p. 460). When the unconscious animal bond representations are brought into consciousness (as in AAI), the "energy becomes serviceable again . . . by humans' conscious attitude towards the collective unconscious" (Jung, 1966, p. 99). This energy activation leads to resolution of trauma symptoms, because dysfunctional boundaries are crossed, leading to emergence of the "transcendent function . . . synonymous with progressive development towards a new attitude" (Jung, 1966, p. 99). EAT can "look like magic, because sometimes you don't understand what has happened . . . between a veteran and the horse. It's like they have a secret language and conversation that only they know" (Blanchette, 2016, p. 3). In other words, this transpersonal explanation highlights the spiritual aspects of PTG, which include making sense of what happened to lead to a larger, more integrated sense of one's self.

Psychophysiological Explanation of AAI Effectiveness

The challenges for traumatized people who develop PTSD include social impairment and avoidance; physiological overarousal; and intrusive thoughts, nightmares, emotions, and flashbacks. In his Polyvagal Theory, Porges (2009; 2011) explains the theoretical basis of these dimensions of trauma along the following lines.

There are three hierarchically operating "phylogenetic response systems" in all mammals that have developed through evolution. The most recent is the mammalian "social engagement system"; farther back is the "mobilization system," or the fight or flight branch of the autonomic nervous system; and the most primitive is the "immobilization system," found in all reptiles, mammals, and amphibians (Porges, 2009, p. 87). This last system is "linked to social communication (e.g., social engagement, facial expression, vocalization, listening)" (Porges, 2009, p. 87). Recruited first, this social engagement system reduces the fight or flight branch's physiological effects and induces calming behaviors by "inhibiting the sympathetic influences on the heart and dampening the hypothalamic–pituitary–adrenal (HPA) axis" (Porges, 2009, p. 87). If this system is unsuccessful in helping the mammal to feel safe, the fight or flight response kicks in and increases metabolic output (e.g., increasing heart rate, raising blood pressure). Then, if this second hierarchical system is also unsuccessful, the third, and most primitive, immobilization system sets in (e.g., feigning death, vasovagal syncope, and behavioral shutdown) by decreasing metabolic input to the point of fainting (Porges, 2009, p. 89).

Which coping strategy or neurophysiological system is being used at any one time depends on whether a person feels safe. Safety is determined by the process of *neuroception*, which Porges (2011) describes as an unconscious process that evaluates subtle voice, face, and movement cues in the environment (p. 11). When the "environment is appraised as being safe, the defensive limbic structures are inhibited, enabling social engagement and calm visceral states to emerge" (Porges, 2009, p. 88).

Increasing Attachment with Neuroception and Prosody

AAI encourages traumatized individuals who may be overusing their mobilization and immobilization systems to begin to feel safer, recruiting the more recently evolved social communication system to return to healthy functioning. Specific aspects of trauma that are less amenable to interactive, verbal, or cognitive forms of person-to-person psychotherapy treatment are apparently more accessible to the nonverbal, tactile dimensions of AAI. Indeed, AAI may be more effective in creating positive outcomes than any particular therapy technique (Furst, 2016), as it offers the opportunity for human-to-animal interactions, which may feel "much safer than dealing with human beings" (Van der Kolk, 2014, p. 215; Tedeschi et al., 2015; Zilcha-Manos, 2017). When AAI is combined with more conventional psychotherapeutic methods, like prolonged exposure (or AAPE, animal-assisted prolonged exposure), or used with trauma-sensitive mindfulness meditation practices (Treleaven, 2018), both of which involve focusing on emotional triggers, animals serve as a kind of "safe place" to prevent retraumatization, by gradually titrating up to spending more time with what is unpleasant. In AAPE, the presence of an animal may reduce the anxiety caused by being in a fearful situation (therapy with another human) or by reexperiencing the fearful memories required in prolonged exposure therapy, especially when the individual is introverted (Lefkowitz et al., 2005). In both treatment practices, animals help individuals feel safe, so that they are not overwhelmed.

Traumatized people also avoid social interactions, because of difficulty discriminating between different emotions that convey anger as opposed to happiness, sadness, and fear (Nazarov et al., 2015). This may reflect inaccurate underlying physiological responses resulting in interpreting the environment as unsafe. In other words, the traumatized person's neuroception, or ability to evaluate relative danger and safety, is faulty (Porges, 2011). Restorative functioning happens in many ways with the help of AAI. Dogs, in particular, provide a compassionate and nonjudgmental connection, with simple physical touch and gaze. They offer emotional attachment and assurance of safety due to their acute hearing and alertness in the environment, encouraging the traumatized person to be "less hypervigilant and have increased success in attempts to reengage in society" (Krause-Parello, Sarni, & Padden, 2016, p. 47). Studies of veterans living with companion dogs report less loneliness, isolation, and worries regarding personal and family safety (Glintborg & Hansen, 2017). In the case of those who are training their own therapy or service animals, owners will need to take them into settings they might otherwise avoid, further decreasing their isolation (Tedeschi et al., 2015) and increasing the sense of "we" referred to earlier.

An important component of neuroception is *prosody*—that is, physiologically soothing vocalizations that people use to talk to their dogs—which can also encourage increased feelings of safety (Porges, 2011). Dogs have a specialized auditory brain center that responds to the human voice, especially a high-pitched one connoting positive affect (Andics et al., 2014); therefore, through learning how to talk with their dogs prosodically—that is, in a tone that "moves back and forth," creating a neuroception of safety (Porges, cited in National Institute for the Clinical Application of Behavioral Medicine, 2016)—traumatized people may learn better how to discriminate positive from negative affect.

The most common empirical studies of using AAI with trauma victims are of those abused as children (O'Haire, Guérin, & Kirkham, 2015). Young people in this category who are in residential care are at particular risk for not accepting conventional therapy methods. "Insecure attachment style, low self-esteem, poor social skills, risk behaviors"—all may make it difficult to bond with treatment staff and therapists" (Muela et al., 2017, p. 1,485). AAI has been particularly effective in reducing depression and anxiety in abused children (Dietz, Davis, & Pennings, 2012), due to their forming a firm attachment with an animal. Observing how the therapist interacts with animals in the session may also instill security and allow traumatized people (especially children) to relax their defenses, feel safe, and experience less emotional numbing, as the trainers are asked to vocalize positive emotions to their dogs (Tedeschi et al., 2015). Furthermore, among sexually abused girls in a group therapy setting, the dog often becomes a safe, nonjudgmental listener, upon which the girls project their feelings; they can also tell their difficult story in the dog's ear, gaining social confidence before telling the group (Reichert, 1994) and reducing sexual concerns (Dietz, Davis, & Pennings, 2012).

When there are multiple animals in a session, for instance, a dog, a hamster, and a parakeet, even more relationship observations can happen, possibly representing different people in the traumatized person's life (Oren & Parish-Plass, 2013). "The cognitive processing of trauma into growth appears to be aided in many people by self-disclosure in supportive social environments" (Tedeschi & Calhoun, 2004, p. 11).

Reducing Psychophysiological Tension through the Oxytocin Link and Love

Several studies have shown that human-animal interactions produce a calming effect upon the many physical correlates of the fight-or-flight neurochemical reactions in the mobilization system (Beetz, Uvnäs-Moberg, Julius, & Kotrschal, 2012; Yount, Ritchie, St. Laurent, Chumley, & Olmert, 2013). If this calming effect is activated, the heart rate slows down and breathing depth is increased. "As a result, we are more calm and relaxed, centered or pleasurably aroused" (Van der Kolk, 2014, p. 83), and may feel less pain due to a "hypnoanalgesia" process (Patterson & Jensen, 2003, p. 505; Engelman, 2013). This calming effect is thought to be due to an increase of endogenous oxytocin (OT) in both animals and humans, much like positive bonding experiences between two humans (Yount et al., 2013). Consequently, when people are feeling safer and calmer, they pay less attention to aversive stimuli, particularly in the form of angry faces (Domes, Steiner, Porges, & Heinrichs, 2013).

OT suppresses neurons "that produce the freezing reaction to fear," social isolation, physical pain, and sleep disturbances, and increases the ability to interpret nonverbal social signals more accurately (Yount et al., 2013, p. 292). One study indicated significant correlations between the OT levels of dogs and their owners, indicating that the levels increased simultaneously in both when owners reported kissing their dogs more (Handlin, Nilssson, Ejdebäck, Hydbring-Sandberg, & Uvnäs-Moberg, 2012). Another study found that, when a dog gazes at its owner, the owner's OT increases, as a manifestation of attachment behavior (Nagasawa, Kikusui, Onaka, & Ohta, 2009), or perhaps love. The "unconditional love" reported between animals and their owners is reflective of Carl Rogers's belief that this condition is a key component in successful psychotherapy (1957).

One veteran AAI initiative called the Warrior Canine Connection (WCC) program enlists wounded veterans in the training of service dogs for fellow veterans. The skills needed by the wounded "trainers" help them regain emotional control, focus their attention, and increase their social competence, interpersonal safety, and sense of well-being (Yount et al., 2013). Throughout the training of the dogs, the veterans' ability to stay mindful of the present moment increases, as they focus on their dogs' behavior in a wide range of situations. In addition, with the added importance of training an animal for other veterans, the "trainers" are able to transcend their own situation and begin to perceive themselves as competent, capable, and nurturing (Lefkowitz et al., 2005). In other words, a spiritual shift takes place within them, resulting in PTG by integrating a more compassionate and effective self-narrative.

> The horses evoke emotions in humans, and in kind, it seems to bring out the best in people. Together, there is something experiential that happens when you can leave a human with a horse. Something happens in the brain and heart, and things start to happen for the greater good (Blanchette, 2016, p. 3).

Speech that combines elements of prosody and linguistic verbal cues, which are socially inviting, can "be as important as touch" in triggering OT release in human beings. This conclusion provides support for why WCC trainers say these positive efforts make them feel better (Seltzer, Ziegler, & Pollak, 2010, p. 2661). EFP has been found to elicit a "calming rush, rather than living with the fight-or-flight feelings" (Nevins et al., 2013, p. 25).

Increasing Groundedness

"Evolutionarily, humans have learned to judge the safety of an environment by the amount of anxiety exhibited by animals," with calm dogs indicating a safe setting (Lefkowitz et al., 2005, p. 278). The presence of a calm animal reminds the owner/patient that, even when flashbacks occur, a threatening situation is no longer present (Yount et al., 2013). AAI decreases this intrusive problem by the integration of mind and body in grounding, wherein dogs respond to a flashback or dissociative situation by nudging, barking, or licking (Krause-Parello, Sarni, & Padden, 2016). This serves as "an alternative object for focus, tactile stimulation or therapeutic distraction for individuals needing assistance, regulating their emotions such as when experiencing sensory overload" (Furst, 2016, p. 55) and decreasing suicide (Altschuler, 2018). During nightmares, dogs may be trained to lick the faces of their persons to wake them up (Weinmeyer, 2015); the results of working with a horse, moreover, may increase one's sleep quality and duration by reducing arousal (Nevins et al., 2013). As traumatized persons are able to re-experience their reality as being safer because of an animal's feedback, they are better able to re-write their narratives and feel their way into a safer world of healthier relationships, leading to PTG (Tedeschi & Calhoun, 2004).

Mindful Observation Leading to Safer Connection and Wholeness

Other studies of trauma have shown that AAI reduces depression, anxiety, stress, and emotional numbing, and encourages staying in the present moment through mindful observation of both horses and dogs (O'Haire, Guérin, & Kirkham, 2015). Being more in the present moment, by observing the effects of one's actions and body language on one's animal, increases mindfulness and creates social awareness in relationships with animals, which can then generalize to humans (Earles, Vernon, & Yetz, 2015). More safely experienced emotional and physiological states may then lead to taking more risks socially with others.

QUALIFICATIONS AND TRAINING REQUIREMENTS

Depending on the specific AAI goals, training is conducted by such organizations as WCC, Pet Partners, and the Certification Board for Equine Interaction Professionals. Having such training and certification, along with following the guidelines set by these organizations, is crucial to conducting AAI efficiently and safely. When accompanied adjunctively by psychotherapy, psychotherapeutic principles and training requirements need to be used, along with a knowledge of animal-welfare principles.

AAI AND DIVERSITY

To avoid cultural stereotyping, one must be sensitive to the inter- and intra-group differences in reactions to AAI; however, few studies have provided "concrete frameworks for how this can be achieved" (Valiyamattam et al., 2018, p. 95). Younger and Latino and African American veterans' retention levels are lowest in conventional treatment for PTSD (Kehle-Forbes & Kimerling, 2017); consequently, these groups may find AAI more useful. In using EFP with the often-overlooked dimension of historical trauma among American Indians, improvements in cultural identity and coping strategies have been shown (Goodkind et al., 2012). Another study indicated that the Japanese, who have numerous AAI programs, view animals as "kin and even assigned a divine status beyond kindship, within the religious context . . . inspiring spirituality" (Valiyamattam et al., 2018, p. 86). Interestingly, despite a lack of evidence-based research using dolphins, dolphin-assisted therapy (DAT) is the "third most common AAI, after canine and equine" in Japan, along with robotic animals (Valiyamattam et al., 2018, p. 88). China has fewer AAI programs than Japan (Valiyamattam et al., 2018, p. 94), but no AAI trauma studies are found in either country. Finally, AAI is a promising nonlanguage-based intervention with multicultural, traumatized refugee children (Every et al., 2017).

SEGMENT OF A CLINICAL VIGNETTE USING AAI

Frank, a shy and reclusive 35-year-old handyman, had been repeatedly sexually assaulted by his uncle throughout much of his life. Frank's physician referred him to my office because he was highly anxious and experiencing severe pain in his shoulders, and found his family situation overwhelming. He feared that setting boundaries with family members would result in rejection. The presence of my therapy dog, CJ, who greeted Frank exuberantly in the waiting room, instantly created a lessening of tension and facilitated Frank's rapport with me. In addition, he noted, "She's so glad to see me—it makes me feel okay!" During the course of nine months, with the help of CJ, a flood of memories from his early life bubbled up in our sessions. These memories reminded him of the love he had felt from his father, as well as his disbelief that he had allowed his uncle to abuse him for years. Frank felt angry that no adult had protected him from this abuse. Frank's heightened physiological arousal at these moments in our session was soothed by petting CJ, and by allowing CJ to lick him whenever he began to dissociate.

One day Frank came to his appointment experiencing unexplained shoulder pain that was "off the scale in intensity." CJ attentively put her paw on Frank's leg as he talked about his pain, and he petted her. When Frank stopped petting CJ and began to express excessive feelings of unworthiness, CJ again put her paw on his leg, to remind him to keep petting her. This served to interrupt the negative spiral of thoughts and "empower" him. As the session progressed into a deeply relaxing episode that included eyes closed and slow-paced breathing, CJ jumped up on the couch and curled up close to Frank. Frank put his hand on CJ, as he listened to my voice leading him through a visualization to reduce his pain. Frank became relaxed, focusing on the "softness of the fur," internalizing this as a visualization of a "soft, warming blanket of deep pink" "engulfing me, giving me strength, helping ease my pain." The combination of the therapy dog's presence, contact, and warmth with the visualization exercise resulted in Frank becoming "100% pain-free" by the end of the session. At home, Frank felt more empowered to set better personal boundaries and assert himself with others.

DISCUSSION AND CONCLUSION

This chapter shows how AAI is an important WPA that leads to transforming trauma through the lens of spirituality. Anecdotal and limited evidence-based literature reviews indicate that AAI offers a complementary, effective intervention, due to animals' unique characteristics, in situations where conventional treatment methods have been unsuccessful.

A holistic paradigm of research that combines shamanic and qualitative, in addition to evidence-based, methods, is called for to better understand the complexities of AAI that facilitate healing. Such a new paradigm must include such unseen factors as one's cultural and spiritual history and beliefs about animals, the therapist's mindset and patient suggestibility factors, and aspects of the setting where AAI takes place. For example, the goals and impact of AAI may vary considerably between, say, the settings of refugee camps and those of military bases. Future research also needs to discern which animal type and breed works best with different types of traumatization, as well as understand when AAI is contraindicated. As national and international research into AAI continues to evolve, comprehensive guiding organizations like IAHAIO may help track and provide a database of this information to advance AAI as a better substantiated, complementary WPA in treating trauma.

REFERENCES

Altschuler, E. (2018). Animal-assisted therapy for posttraumatic stress disorder: Lessons from "case reports" in media stories. *Military Medicine*, *183*, 11–13. doi: 10.1093/milmed/usx073.

Andics, A., Gácsi, M., Faragó, T., Kis, A., & Miklósi, A. (2014). Voice-sensitive regions in the dog and human brain are revealed by comparative FMRI. *Cell Symposia*, *24*(5), 574–78. doi: 10.1016/j.cub.2014.01.058.

Beetz, A., Uvnäs-Moberg, K., Julius, H., & Kotrschal, K. (2012). Psychosocial and psychophysiological effects of human–animal interactions: The possible role of oxytocin. *Frontiers in Psychology*, *3*, 234–45. doi: 10.3389/fpsyg.2012.00234.

Blanchette, D. (2016). Equine therapy eases veterans' symptoms of PTSD. *Wall Street Journal*. Retrieved from http://www.sj-r.com/news/20161110/equine-therapy-eases-veterans-symptoms-of-ptsd.

Carminati, G., Lehotkay, R., Martin, F., & Carminati, F. (2013). A hypothesis about Jung's collective unconscious and animal-assisted therapy. *NeuroQuantology*, *11*(3), 451–65. doi: 10.14704/nq.2013.11.3.679.

Dalai Lama. (2011). *Beyond religion: Ethics for a whole world*. New York: Houghton-Mifflin Harcourt.

Dietz, T. J., Davis, D., & Pennings, J. (2012). Evaluating animal-assisted therapy in group treatment for child sexual abuse. *Journal of Child Sexual Abuse*, *21*, 665–83. doi: 10:1080/10538712.2012.726700.

Domes, G., Steiner, A., Porges, S. W., & Heinrichs, M. (2013). Oxytocin differentially modulates eye gaze to naturalistic social signs of happiness and anger. *Psychoneuro-endocrinology*, *38*(7), 1,198–1,202. doi: 10.1016lj.psyneven.2012.10.002.

Earles, J. L., Vernon, L. L., & Yetz, J. P. (2015). Equine-assisted therapy for anxiety and posttraumatic stress symptoms. *Journal of Traumatic Stress*, *28*, 149–52. doi: 10.1002/jts.21990.

Eliade, M. (1964). *Shamanism: Archaic techniques of ecstasy*. Princeton, NJ: Princeton University Press.

Engelman, S. (2013). Palliative care and animal-assisted therapy. *Omega: Journal of Death and Dying*, *67*(1/2), 63–67. doi: 10.2190/OM.67.1-2g.

Every, D., Smith, K., Smith, B., Trigg, J., & Thompson, K. (2017). How can a donkey fly on the plane? The benefits and limits of animal therapy with refugees. *Clinical Psychologist*, 21, 44–53. doi: 10.1111/cp.12071.

Furst, G. (2016). Helping war veterans with posttraumatic stress disorder: Incarcerated individuals' role in therapeutic animal programs. *Journal of Psychosocial Nursing Mental Health Service*, *54*(5), 49–57. doi: 10:3928/0279369520160420-07.

Goodkind, J., LaNoue, M., Lee, C., Freeland, L., & Freund, R. (2012). Feasibility, acceptability, and initial findings from a community-based cultural mental health intervention for American Indian youth and their families. *Journal of Community Psychology*, *40*(4), 381–405. doi: 10.1002/jcop.20517.

Glintborg, C., & Hansen, T. G. (2017). How are service dogs for adults with posttraumatic stress disorder integrated with rehabilitation in Denmark? A case study. *Animals*, *7*, 33. doi: 10.3390/ani7050033.

Grob, C. (1994). Psychiatric research with hallucinogens: What have we learned? *Yearbook for Ethnomedicine and the Study of Consciousness*. Retrieved from www.druglibrary.org/schaffer/lsd/grob.htm.

Handlin, L., Nilsson, A., Edjebäck, M., Hydbring-Sandberg, E., & Uvnäs-Moberg, K. (2012). Associations between the psychological characteristics of the human–dog relationship and oxytocin and cortisol levels. *Anthro2005*, *25*(2), 215–28. doi: 10.2752/175303712x13316289505468.

Hoagwood, K., Acri, M., Morrissey, M., & Peth-Pierce, R. (2017). Animal-assisted therapies for youth with or at risk for mental health problems: A systematic review. *Applied Developmental Science*, *21*(1), 1–13. doi: 10.1080/1088691.2015.1145267.

Hundt, N. E., Helm, A., Smith, T. L., Lamkin, J., Cully, J. A., & Stanley, M. A. (2017, December). Failure to engage: A qualitative study of veterans who decline evidence-based psychotherapies for PTSD. *Psychological Services*, 1–7. doi: 10.1037/ser0000212.

International Association of Human–Animal Interactions Organization (IAHAIO). (2014). *The IAHAIO definitions for animal assisted activity and guidelines for wellness of animals involved*. White paper. Retrieved from https://petpartners.org/wp-content/uploads/2015/07/8000IAHAIO-WHITE-PAPER-TASK-FORCE-FINAL-REPORT-070714.pdf.

Jung, C. G. (1966). The archetypes of the collective unconscious. In H. Read, M. Fordham, G. Adler, & W. McGuire (eds.), *Two essays on analytical psychology* (pp. 90–113). Princeton, NJ: Princeton University Press.

Kabat-Zinn, J. (1994). *Wherever you go, there you are: Mindfulness meditation in everyday life*. New York: Hyperion.

Kehle-Forbes, S., & Kimerling, R. (2017). Patient engagement in PTSD treatment. *PTSD Research Quarterly*, *28*(30), 1–4.

Knobloch-Bollmann, H. S., Charlet, A., Hoffmann, L. C., Eliava, M., Khrulev, S., & Grinevich, V. (2012). Evoked axonal oxytocin release in central amygdala attenuates fear response. *Neuron*, *73*(3), 553–66. doi: 10.1016/j.neuron.2011.11.030.

Krause-Parello, C., Sarni, S., & Padden, E. (2016). Military veterans and canine assistance for posttraumatic stress disorder: A narrative review of the literature. *Nurse Education Today*, *47*, 43–50. doi: 10.1016/j.nedt.2016.04.020.

Lefkowitz, C., Prout, M., Bleiberg, J., Paharia, I., & Debiak, D. (2005). Animal-assisted prolonged exposure: A treatment for survivors of sexual assault suffering from posttraumatic stress disorder. *Society and Animals*, *13*, 275–95.

Levinson, B. (1969). *Pet-oriented child psychotherapy*. Springfield, IL: Thomas.

Lundqvist, M., Carlsson, P., Sjödahl, R., Theodorsson, E., & Levin, L. (2017). Patient benefit of dog-assisted interventions in health care: A systematic review. *Bio-Med Central Complementary and Alternative Medicine*, *117*(358), 1–12. doi: 10.11861512906-017-1844-7.

Mormann, F., Dubois, J., Kornblith, S., Milosavljevc, M., Cerf, M., Tsuchiya, N., & Koch, C. (2012). A category-specific response to animals in the right human amygdala. *Nature Neuroscience*, *14*(10), 1,247–49. doi: 10.1038/nn.2899.

Muela, A., Balluerka, N., Amiano, N., Caldentey, M. A., & Aliri, J. (2017). Animal-assisted psychotherapy for young people with behavioral problems in residential care. *Clinical Psychology and Psychotherapy*, *24*, 1,485–94. doi: 10.1002/cpp.2112.

Nagasawa, M., Kikusui, T., Onaka, T., & Ohta, M. (2009). Dog's gaze at its owner increases owner's urinary oxytocin during social interaction. *Hormones and Behavior*, *55*, 434–41. doi: 10.1016/j.yhbeh.2008.12.002.

National Institute for the Clinical Application of Behavioral Medicine (Producer). (2016). *How to use polyvagal theory to help patients "reset" the nervous system after trauma*. Transcript of Part 1, Webinar. Storrs, CT: NICABM.

Nazarov, A., Frewen, P., Oremus, C., Schellenberg, E., McKinnon, M., & Lanius, R. (2015). Comprehension of affective prosody in women with posttraumatic stress disorder related to childhood abuse. *Acta Psychiatrica Scandinavica*, *131*, 342–49. doi: 10.1111/acps.12364.

Nevins, R., Finch, S., Hickling, E., & Barnett, S. (2013). The Saratoga WarHorse project: A case study of the treatment of psychological distress in a veteran of Operation Iraqi Freedom. *Advances*, *27*(4), 22–25.

O'Haire, M. E., & Rodriguez, K. E. (2018). Preliminary efficacy of service dogs as a complementary treatment for posttraumatic stress disorder in military members and veterans. *Journal of Consulting and Clinical Psychology*, *86*(2),179–88. doi: 10.1037/cep0000267.

O'Haire, M. E., Guérin, N. A., & Kirkham, A. C. (2015). Animal-assisted intervention for trauma: A systematic literature review. *Frontiers in Psychology*, *6*(1,121), 1–16. doi: 10.3389/fpsyg.2015.01121.

Oren, D., & Parish-Plass, N. (2013). The integration of animals into the therapy process and its implications as a unique medium in psychotherapy. In N. Parish-Plass (ed.), *Animal-assisted psychotherapy: Theory, issues, and practice* (pp. 3–45). Lafayette, IN: Purdue University Press.

Patterson, D., & Jensen, M. (2003). Hypnosis and pain. *Psychological Bulletin*, *129*(4), 495–521. doi: 10.1037/0033-2909.129.4.495.

Porges, S. W. (2009). The polyvagal theory: New insights into adaptive reactions of the autonomic nervous system. *Cleveland Clinic Journal of Medicine*, *76*(2), s86–s90. doi: 10.3949/ccjm.76s2.17.

Porges, S. W. (2011). *The polyvagal theory: Neurophysiological foundations of emotions, attachment, communication, self-regulation*. New York: W. W. Norton.

Reichert, E. (1994). Play and animal-assisted therapy: A group treatment model for sexually abused girls ages 9–13. *Family Therapy*, *2*(1), 55–62.

Rogers, C. (1957). The necessary and sufficient conditions of therapeutic personality change. *Journal of Consulting and Clinical Psychology*, *21*(2), 95–103.

Saunders, G., Biswas, K., Serpi, T., McGovern, S., Groer, S., & Fallon, M. (2017). Design and challenges for a randomized, multisite clinical trial comparing the use of service dogs and emotional support dogs in veterans with posttraumatic stress disorder (PTSD). *Contemporary Clinical Trials*, *62*, 105–13. doi: 10.1016/j.cct.2017.08.017.

Seltzer, L. J., Ziegler, T. E., & Pollak, S. D. (2010). Social vocalizations can release oxytocin in humans. *Proceedings of the Royal Society, B: Biological Sciences*. doi: 10.1098/rspb.2010.0567.

Seymour, V. (2016). The human–nature relationship and its impact on health: A critical review. *Frontiers in Public Health*, *4*, 260. doi: 10.3389/fpubn.2016.00260.

Siegel, D. (2010). *The mindful therapist*. New York: W. W. Norton.

Staudt, M., & Cherry, D. (2017). Equine-facilitated therapy and trauma: Current knowledge, future needs. *Advances in Social Work*, *18*(1), 403–14. doi: 10.18060/21292.

Tedeschi, P., Sisa, M., Olmert, M. D., Parish-Plass, N., & Yount, R. (2015). Treating human trauma with the help of animals: Trauma-informed intervention for child maltreatment and adult posttraumatic stress. In A. H. Fine (ed.), *Handbook on animal-assisted therapy: Theoretical foundations and guidelines for animal-assisted interventions* (pp. 305–19). San Diego, CA: Academic Press. doi: 10.1016/B978-0-12-8-1292-5.00022.5.

Tedeschi, R. G., & Calhoun, L. G. (2004). Posttraumatic growth: Conceptual foundations and empirical evidence. *Psychological Inquiry*, *15*(1), 1–18. doi: 10.1207/s15327965pli150101.

Treleaven, D. (2018). *Trauma-sensitive mindfulness: Practices for safe and transformative healing*. Kindle Edition. New York: W. W. Norton.

U.S. Department of Justice. (2011). *ADA requirements: Service animals*. Retrieved from https://www.ada.gov/service_animals_2010.htm.

Van der Kolk, B. (2014). *The body keeps the score*. New York: Penguin.

Valiyamattam, G., Yamamoto, M., Fanucchi, L., & Wang, F. (2018). Multicultural considerations in animal-assisted interventions. *Human-Animal Interaction Bulletin*, *6*, 82–104. doi : 10.1016/j.sbspro.2013.04.343.

Weinmeyer, R. (2015). Service dogs for veterans with posttraumatic stress disorder. *American Medical Association Journal of Ethics*, *17*(6), 54752. doi: 10.1001/journal of ethics.2015.17.6. hlaw1-1506.

Wilson, E. O. (1984). *Biophilia*. Cambridge, MA: Harvard University Press.

Yount, R., Ritchie, E. C., St. Laurent, M., Chumley, P., & Olmert, M. D. (2013). The role of service dog training in the treatment of combat-related PTSD. *Psychiatric Annals*, *43*(6), 292–95. doi: 10.3928/00485713-20130606-11.

Zilcha-Manos, S. (2017). Resolution of alliance ruptures: The special case of animal-assisted psychotherapy. *Clinical Child Psychology and Psychiatry*, *22*(1), 34–45. doi: 10.177/1359104516671385.

Chapter Seven

The Therapeutic Spiral Model

A Psychodramatic Whole-Person Approach for Working with Trauma

Sylvia Israel

The Therapeutic Spiral Model (TSM) is a clinically modified psychodramatic approach for working with people who have experienced trauma. J. L. Moreno—physician, psychiatrist, and father of psychodrama—rejected psychology's embrace of the stern medical model, which views people through the lens of illness or pathology with the goal of symptom reduction. Instead, Moreno treated the whole person, integrating psychology, psychiatry, medicine, and social work, along with seeing people with unique experiences, points of view, spirituality, and dreams in the context of their communities. In *Who Shall Survive* (1953), Moreno asserts his broad vision of healing: "A truly therapeutic procedure cannot have less an objective than the whole of mankind" (p. 3). Emphasizing creativity, spontaneity, and the importance of encountering people where they are in the present, he created a therapeutic theater model in which all people were welcome and every aspect of one's life could be explored, honored, and engaged. In a psychodrama, he would have the protagonists (or clients) enact roles—physically, emotionally, and cognitively—thereby developing the capacity to be with the entirety of their experiences. These shared role-plays helped participants connect with the deepest parts of themselves and with each other.

Zerka Moreno, his wife and the mother of psychodrama, affirmed that actively sharing internal experiences through words or actions is particularly useful for trauma survivors who often may be trying to hide their internal chaos. By externalizing thoughts, feelings, defenses, and behaviors, they can view them from a place of observation, interact and play with them, and begin to make changes (Z. T. Moreno, Blomkvist, & Rützel, 2000).

In 1992, when they were leading psychodrama groups with trauma survivors, Kate Hudgins and Francesca Toscani observed that participants were at risk for retraumatization through intense affects and uncontrolled regressions when enacting or witnessing traumatic scenes. This led them to shift their lens from the interpersonal realm of psychodrama to an internal focus on self-organization. Drawing on Moreno's *social atom* (J. L. Moreno, 1953), which is a map of the interpersonal relationships in one's life, Toscani and Hudgins (1995) created the Trauma Survivor's Intrapsychic Role Atom (TSIRA), an internal role atom and the cornerstone of the TSM. The TSIRA offers a map that provides a framework for working with trauma survivors, emphasizing safety, containment, and strengths (Hudgins, 2001, 2017; Hudgins & Toscani, 2013). The TSIRA includes clinically modified psychodrama interventions to work with internal roles needed for healing and posttraumatic growth (PTG) following the experience of trauma.

In the past 25 years, TSM has been used in more than 40 countries (Hudgins, 2017). For example, TSM counselors worked with the 3rd Military Division of the Chinese Army to help survivors of the 2008 earthquake. In Australia, TSM practitioners provided training for refugee counselors at the NSW New Service for Treatment and Rehabilitation of Torture and Trauma Survivors. In South Africa, TSM counselors worked with a racially mixed group of African tribal leaders and immigrant social workers brought together by the South African nonprofit Acting thru "Ukubuyiselwa"—a Zulu word for regaining dignity. TSM trainers worked with leaders, teachers, social workers, and families living in an active war zone in Palestine. TSM practitioners, along with other psychodramatists, worked with the community in Charlottesville, Virginia, after the racial violence in 2017. There are more than 1,000 people who have received benefits from being introduced to the TSM by trainers in Australia, Indonesia, Canada, China, Egypt, England, Germany, South Africa, Taiwan, and the United States.

In this chapter, we present an overview of the research on TSM followed by a detailed description and application of the TSIRA. Case examples are included to demonstrate using the TSIRA in practice with people who have experienced trauma. Our intention is that clinicians from a wide range of theoretical orientations should find the TSIRA to be a useful guide in conceptualizing the healing process of trauma survivors, as well as a map for treatment for individuals and groups. We hope that this tool provides another lens from which to view traumatized clients as whole people, with the capacity to grow and change, and develop new roles by accessing their spontaneity and creativity.

EVIDENCE-BASED RESEARCH AND THEORETICAL INTEGRATION OF THE TSM

TSM is anchored in the research and theories of psychodrama and experiential therapy, as well as those of clinical psychology related to trauma and attachment, and advances in neuroscience of the brain and human interaction (Giacomucci, 2019; Hug, 2013). Baim (2013) and Wieser (2011) detail the most up-to-date research on the use and effectiveness of psychodrama across settings from education to therapy, and from small groups to large cultural entities. Stadler, Wieser, and Kirk (2016) demonstrate psychodrama's effectiveness across various settings, populations, languages, and cultures. Rezacian, Mazumdar, and Sen (1997), conducting a comparison study on depression, found that psychodrama was more effective than a standard talk-therapy psychiatric group. Greenberg, Watson, and Lietaer (1998) show that experiential psychotherapy was equally as effective as psychodynamic and cognitive behavioral therapies, and more effective with people who had experienced trauma. Hudgins and Kiesler (1987) integrate Gestalt therapy (Perls, Hefferline, & Goodman, 1951) and focusing (Gendlin, 1957) with psychodramatic doubling in a quantitative study, placing TSM psychodrama into the research on experiential therapy. Greenberg (2013) summarizes the research on experiential therapies, including psychodrama and TSM, inside the broader psychological literature, concluding that TSM shows great promise in effectiveness.

Quantitative research on TSM's Containing Double (described later in this chapter) showed statistically significant decreases in dissociation, depression, anxiety, and general symptoms of PTSD during a six-month follow-up after three individual therapy sessions (Hudgins & Drucker, 1998; Hudgins, Drucker, & Metcalf, 2000). McVea and Gow (2006) detail the importance of the role of auxiliaries in the TSM. Hudgins, Culbertson, and Hug (2009) show TSM's effectiveness when combined with literature, music, and public speaking in leadership training in the community following episodes of violence. Perry et al. (2016) demonstrate that the TSM action protocol for a three-day weekend produced increases in self-esteem and connection for military women who had served in Afghanistan and Iraq. Additional research is being conducted in Taiwan, Egypt, and the United States.

Neurobiological research has shown that experiential methods are the treatment of choice for trauma prevention and repair (Cozolino, 2016; Siegel, 2010), emphasizing the constant interaction of interpersonal experiences related to biological and social factors (Cozolino, 2002, 2014; Siegel, 2007). The clinical model of TSM developed separately but concurrently with research on the neurobiology of trauma and interpersonal affective neurobiology (Panksepp, 1998; Siegel, 2012). State-of-the-art fMRIs have shown that the brain is an ever-changing organization of neural networks, synaptic connections, and molecular changes, as it interacts with the here and now of internal states and interpersonal relationships (Cozolino, 2016). Hudgins demonstrates that, as trauma survivors safely experience the roles of the TSIRA, their neurobiology changes, thereby creating a new level of self-organization (2007). As clients integrate the Containing Double, their ability to balance thinking and feeling expands. Embodying the Body Double reduces dissociation. Once resourced with prescribed strength roles, clients demonstrate increased spontaneity.

A CLINICAL MAP FOR TRAUMA: THE TRAUMA SURVIVOR'S INTERNAL ROLE ATOM (TSIRA)

Moreno's spontaneity and creativity theory is at the core of TSM and psychodrama. He defines *spontaneity* as having an adequate response to a novel situation or a new response to an old one (J. L. Moreno, 1953). Moreno's role theory conceptualizes the self as being a sum of all the roles we play, with our spontaneity and creativity making it possible to expand our repertoire of roles. TSM followed up by creating an internal role map, the TSIRA, as a template or guide for therapists and clients to make sense of the internal and often chaotic reality of a trauma survivor's self-presentation. When trauma happens, survival modes of coping—for example, fight, flight, or freeze—lock into both neurobiological and social roles, thus inhibiting the development of spontaneous and creative actions. TSM, using the TSIRA, seeks to create new narratives based on corrective emotional experiences and changes in internal roles to create PTG (Hudgins, 2015). It is most useful to talk about problems and situations in terms of the roles being played, because the terminology is relatively familiar and nonpathologizing.

The TSIRA details a three-stage process model of trauma-informed experiential change (Hudgins, Culbertson, & Hug, 2009). Stage 1 presents prescriptive roles that focus on developing the ability for nonjudgmental observation, strengths, and containment. Stage 2 uses the TSM Trauma Triangle of Victim, Perpetrator, and Abandoning Authority to visualize the roles that are internalized from trauma. Stage 3 evidences the emergence of transformational roles as a result of the interaction of the prescriptive and trauma-based roles.

Stage 1: Prescriptive Roles and Functions: Observation, Restoration/ Strengths, and Containment

Without new resources, trauma survivors risk retraumatization when confronting past experiences. Thus, roles are prescribed to decrease affect and increase cognitive functioning, much like a psychiatrist prescribes medication. The seven prescribed roles prevent retraumatization and keep protagonists/clients in their window of tolerance. As presented in table 7.1, the function of observation is contained in the Observing Ego; the function of restoration or strengths is held by intrapsychic, interpersonal, and transpersonal roles; and the function of containment is held by the Containing Double (CD), Body Double (BD), and Manager of Defenses (MD).

Prescriptive Role of Observation

The first prescriptive internal role that is concretized to establish a cognitive part of self-awareness is the Observing Ego (OE). To change, people need to be able to observe the whole of who they are—relationships, behaviors, thoughts, and emotions—neutrally and without judgment, shame, or blame. This might appear to be simple, but a trauma survivor's internal self-organization is often filled with negative messages, horrific images, unmanaged affect, and chaotic or nonexistent relationships, which make it difficult to maintain an accurate and neutral record of what is happening at a behavioral and interpersonal level. In the role of OE, clients are able to expand their window of tolerance and sustain the emotional distance necessary for self-compassion that leads to healing. In the session, therapists may have clients choose an inspirational card featuring an animal, a flower, the Buddha, etc., to represent the energy and strength that supports them, keeping them in the OE role.

As an illustration, Sally, a woman in her 40s, was angry with her husband Bob, because he would not stand up to his mother on her behalf after Sally and his mother had a disagreement. In a drama, Sally acknowledged that she was stuck in the belief that Bob's mother was his priority. Sally chose an inspirational card of a redwood tree to support her and embody the role of OE, sharing, "Redwood trees have been on Earth thousands of years. I am sure they have witnessed many struggles in relationships. This tree is very tall and can get a good perspective, which is what I need." As Sally took the role of OE, she moved across the room to where she had placed the redwood tree card so she could see the situation from that perspective and with that

Table 7.1. Prescriptive Roles and Functions

Roles	Function
Observing Ego (OE)	observation
intrapsychic/personal strength interpersonal strength transpersonal/spiritual strength	restoration/strengths
Containing Double (CD) Body Double (BD) Manager of Defenses (MD)	containment

strength. She stood taller with feet planted on the floor and spoke in the first-person role of an internalized strength, stating,

> I see that I am feeling hurt and abandoned, the same way as when I was seven and we moved 3,000 miles away. My parents never talked about the move with me. At eight, my father left the family, and I became my mother's caretaker and confidante. I can see from this position that I am on the lookout for any hint of Bob siding with his mother. This makes me angry, and I lash out at Bob, and then he withdraws. I also observe that Bob's relationship with me is his priority, and that he is setting limits with his mother.

Leaving the role of OE, Sally felt calm and centered. She now knew more clearly that she had work to do on her earlier wounding, so she could do her part in creating the loving relationship she wanted.

Prescriptive Roles of Restoration/Strengths

For restoration, or to reclaim lost spontaneity, people need to draw on intrapsychic, interpersonal, and transpersonal strengths to gain resilience. Since many trauma survivors isolate themselves and rely on their own skills for survival, helping them to identify, acknowledge, and embody strengths on which they have relied or which they have developed since the trauma is both affirming and healing. *Intrapsychic* strengths, like perseverance, courage, optimism, and stubbornness, are roles that are present within the individual. *Interpersonal* strengths refer to caring people (or animals) that are supportive resources for healing work, for instance, family members, ancestors, teachers, pets, or even an inspiring author. Positive interpersonal roles reinforce attachment and encourage brain plasticity (Badenoch, 2008). The trauma survivor needs the power of a transpersonal strength to confront the perpetrator and other trauma-based roles. Transpersonal (beyond human) strengths can be as varied as human cultures and can include Jesus, the Buddha, nature, music, and so on. We present an example of how embodying the role of a spiritual teacher (both an interpersonal and a transpersonal strength) may guide clients to finding a new way of being.

Jane, the protagonist in a group psychodrama session, shared that she had recently expressed extreme anger at her 12-year-old son when, at a large family gathering, he said that he would not sit at the children's table if there were young children present. When Jane "sculpted" how she felt (a psychodrama term for placing people in positions that express the inner world), she took the body position of someone ready to attack physically, raising her arm high. To encapsulate how she felt, she said, "I want to kill you." Taking the role of her son, she showed him backing away from her, arms raised in a defensive position, and stating, "Get away from me." Jane was aware of childhood trauma resulting from her mother's rage when she did not behave as expected. As Jane watched group members enact her sculpture, she knew she was caught in the trauma roles but could not find her way out. It was only through inviting her spiritual teacher, the Buddhist Monk Thich Nhat Hanh, to help her that she was able to move forward. The director took time guiding Jane to embody fully the role of Thich Nhat Hanh, establishing what he was wearing, how he stood, how he breathed, and so forth. As Jane slowly stepped into the role and took on his mannerisms, her breath and speech slowed. A hush came over the group, as the energy in the room softened. In this role, Jane told herself, "Breathe. Breathe and smile. There is no need to fear your thoughts or feelings. Embrace them. Smile at yourself and at your son. Breathing in, you are peaceful; breathing out, you are calm." Jane found the peace, acceptance, and guidance that she was seeking. Integrating these Buddhist teachings, Jane returned to the original scene and approached her son as a wise mother with an open, loving heart. Jane could now hear her son's request, open her arms, and embrace him. With the help of the group, she laughed, as she realized that his desire to not be at the table with younger children was age-appropriate.

Prescriptive Roles of Containment

One of the most devastating after-effects of trauma is an inability to self-regulate and experience life within the window of tolerance. Trauma survivors can easily become overwhelmed by emotional triggers at unpredictable moments and regress or dissociate. People who have experienced violence have, in fact, felt horror, terror, rage, grief, helplessness, and despair. It can often be dangerous to cry out in pain or express any feeling at the time of trauma, so these intense feelings become dissociated and are held outside of psychological awareness, until they break into everyday consciousness.

The TSIRA describes three roles of containment: the Containing Double (CD) (Hudgins & Toscani, 2013), the Body Double (BD) (Burden & Ciotola, 2002; Carnabucci & Ciotola, 2013), and the Manager of Defenses (MD) (Hudgins & Toscani, 2013). Here the focus is on increasing self-regulation and containment of dissociation, emotional volatility, and the rigid but necessary defenses that follow trauma. The roles of containment titrate the emotions into measurable dosages to help clients stay in the window of tolerance.

In psychodrama, the Double gives voice to the inner reality of the client/protagonist, expressing what is *not said*, expanding unconscious awareness and increasing emotions. It is described as echoing the symbiotic stage of child development, when the caretaker knows exactly what the baby is experiencing and puts words to what is unspoken. TSM delineates two specific doubling roles that are useful with trauma survivors. The most used structure of the TSIRA, the Containing Double (CD), is an inner voice that helps guide the trauma survivor toward spontaneity and creativity by balancing thinking and feeling. Acting like the brain's corpus callosum, the CD helps exchange information commonly stored in the right hemisphere of the brain (emotions, sensations, and images) with the left side (words, numbers, and language). As in psychodrama, the CD assumes the same posture and gestures as the client, standing slightly behind, where s/he can see the client's affect. The Double speaks in an "I" voice, and the client is instructed to repeat what was correct or change what was said to make it accurate. The CD speaks slowly and sensitively, pacing oneself so as to establish an empathic bond and gently hold, contain, and lead the client. In an individual session, the therapist may choose to take the role of the CD for a portion of a session or even an entire session. In a group, a group member or trained assistant takes on the role.

The Body Double (BD) contains, calms, and soothes the body, if feelings start to become overwhelming and the cognitive and emotional container of the CD is not enough. The BD creates a safe, grounding, embodied experience for people who suffer from trauma, as well as eating and dissociative identity disorders. The BD picks up on such autonomic experiences as facial expressions, breathing, and proprioception. It teaches clients to calm the amygdala and establish a sense of safety in their bodies. While the CD and BD are demarcated in their specific purposes, they are often played as one role.

Finally, the Manager of Defenses (MD) is a role that is clinically necessary when clients begin to demonstrate psychological defenses preventing them from doing their healing work. Defenses are honored for their help with survival and maintaining safety in the past. Clients are invited to consider if defenses are needed as they do their healing work in the present. The roles of containment are demonstrated in the following vignette: Sam demonstrates signs of dissociation as he begins his drama with the stated goal of speaking lovingly to his younger self. The director invites Sam to choose someone to play his CD and BD (as one role). The CD/BD stands beside Sam and says,

> I can take a deep breath and stay present. When I notice myself dissociating, I can feel the four corners of my feet on the floor. I can feel the support of the Earth. When I am ready, I can look up and see the people here supporting me to do the work I came here for. I can take one step toward that work now.

Sam then chooses a white scarf to represent dissociation. He invites a group member who he describes as "grounded" to be the MD and hold the dissociation scarf. Sam places his MD across the room and says, "When I see you with my dissociation, I will remember to ground myself." With his CD and his strength roles, Sam returns to the scene of speaking lovingly to his younger self.

Stage 2: Roles—The Trauma Triangle

The Trauma Triangle is a simple, nonpathologizing, clinical action structure representing a closed circuit of energy embedded in the self-organization and neurobiology of those who have survived trauma. It consists of three trauma-based roles: victim, perpetrator, and abandoning authority (Hudgins & Toscani, 2013; Toscani & Hudgins, 1995). These roles, while distinct in their meanings and psychological functions, collaborate in trapping trauma survivors into a destructive cycle of repetition. Although the roles began in response to hurtful and traumatic situations, clients quickly see how they are now internalized and how the pattern plays out in their current relationships. There is often a sense of relief as the pattern they have been stuck in is concretized and even normalized as occurring with everyone with unresolved trauma. Trauma survivors also become hopeful as they see that they can break the pattern of repetitive energy going nowhere by developing new spontaneous and creative roles (as demonstrated in stage 3), thus removing themselves from the Triangle.

In the victim role, clients hold and communicate the story and experience of the trauma. When clients are triggered and feel like helpless children, they are displaying the effects of unprocessed, often intense and dissociated, feelings of horror, terror, rage, grief, and despair. These feelings, which could not be experienced at the time of trauma, are unconsciously stored in the limbic system, keeping the clients stuck in the past. The conscious reexperiencing of the victim role enables clients to transform the role to that of the wounded child, who has suffered greatly and is in need of care and compassion.

The psychological function of the perpetrator role is to keep the trauma out of consciousness. Images of the past drive this role internally, but, rather than taking the victim role, the self organizes around an illusory sense of power and begins to repeat patterns of violence, blame, and shame toward the self and/or others. This can be experienced as hearing a critical voice saying that they are bad, worthless, or crazy; experiencing fragmented, intrusive images and sensations; and suffering disturbing body memories and flashbacks. Identifying with the role of perpetrator can feel powerful and life-saving following trauma. Individuals, groups, societies, and even cultures

Table 7.2. Trauma-Based Roles and Functions

Role	Function
victim	communication of trauma
perpetrator	keep trauma out of consciousness
abandoning authority	show what was lacking at time of original trauma

can live in a chronic state of perpetration, disguising their own feelings of victimization and fear. Learning to accept the perpetrator role is necessary to understand fully the impact of trauma on self-organization.

The psychological function of the abandoning authority is to show what was lacking in previous attempts to help. Trauma can only happen when authority figures abandon their role to stop abuse, neglect, or oppression. The abandoning authority role is internalized when there was no rescuer available in the interpersonal world, an experience that leads trauma survivors to abandon themselves to dissociation, self-harm, addictions, eating disorders, and lack of self-care, as well as suicide attempts and, at worst, successful suicides. When clients hear the negative voices of the perpetrator or feel the despair of the victim role, they ignore them and feel powerless to intervene. Experiencing this role can provide clients with information about the original disruption in attachment. The clinical goal is for clients to move off the Trauma Triangle by developing the transformative role of appropriate authority.

The vignette that follows demonstrates a client walking the Trauma Triangle, an important step on the path to healing. The therapist begins by writing each role on a separate piece of paper, placing the papers on the floor at each point of a triangle, and explaining what each role represents. In an individual session, the Triangle is often placed within a circle of scarves that represent the strengths of the client.

Lita chooses group members to play her prescriptive roles: courage and creativity (intrapsychic), her wife Sandy and her aunt Molly (interpersonal), the goddess and nature (transpersonal), the role of OE (observation), and her CD (containment). Lita enters the Triangle at the victim role. She identifies that, when she is overwhelmed, she feels numb, frozen, and dissociated. Standing at the victim role corner, she says, “I am bad. There is something wrong with me. I don’t deserve to be loved.” Lita describes how, as a child, she felt ashamed when her father would go out drinking and forget to pick her up from school, leave her alone at home for hours or days, and hit and berate her. Moving to the perpetrator role, she states, “Why don’t you behave? There is something wrong with you. You need to do better. You are bad.” In the role of abandoning authority, Lita turns her back on the victim and perpetrator. She feels helpless, weak, and somewhat dissociated, as she says, “I don’t see a problem. There is nothing I can do. This is how it is and always will be.” Lita names this as the role both her parents played. Her father completely abandoned his authority, even at times being unable to provide basic necessities. Her mother did not protect her and even allowed her father to have sole custody when, after divorcing, she emigrated to another country. Lita sees how this pattern lives inside of her, in her physiology—in her brain and body. She wants to take the next step (stage 3) and move off the Trauma Triangle.

Stage 3: Transformation—Posttraumatic Growth

The TSIRA concretizes several transformative roles that develop naturally, as the prescriptive roles interact with the trauma-based roles for the final stage of trauma repair and PTG. These TSIRA-delineated roles add a more detailed and observable definition of PTG to the literature. Calhoun and Tedeschi (2014), who describe PTG as the positive changes that often occur as a result of struggling with a traumatic event, have observed them across six categories of change. The TSIRA has concretized these changes into such transformative roles as sleeping-awakening child, various good-enough roles, and the appropriate and ultimate authority roles. The organic emergence of transformative roles puts into action the idea of the innate ancient wisdom of the human spirit that brings healing (Z. T. Moreno, Horvatin, & Schreiber, 2006).

The sleeping-awakening child role is the part of the self that holds intact the trauma survivor's innocence, creativity, spontaneity, and inherent goodness. These parts were never lost; they simply went to sleep and stayed protected at the time of the trauma through dissociation and other defenses. Clients are happy and relieved to acknowledge this role, knowing that there is a part of themsleves that was unaffected by the trauma. It is a wonderful moment when the client has created enough safety that this role awakens naturally.

Trauma causes disruptions in attachment to others. Corrective scenes of developmental repair with good-enough interpersonal experiences are internalized into self-organization and the ever-changing experiential brain. TSM dramas include scenes in which one or more roles—the good-enough parent, good-enough significant other, and good-enough spirituality—are present. Through actual experiences of hearing a comforting voice, being held safely while crying, testing out new boundaries, or receiving wise guidance, clients can internalize new experiences.

Table 7.3. Transformation Roles and Functions

Roles	Function
sleeping-awakening child change agent manager of healthy defenses	autonomy
good-enough parent good-enough significant other good-enough spirituality	
appropriate authority ultimate authority	integration

The appropriate authority role was developed in contradiction to the abandoning authority role. The appropriate authority role can maintain boundaries to stop trauma from occurring, as well as nurture the wounded child. This role often emerges naturally in a drama to break up the internalized pattern of the Trauma Triangle. When the appropriate authority is integrated and in charge of self-organization, it is one small, yet profound, step to the final TSM transformative role of ultimate authority. After integrating and feeling secure in the positive roles of the TSIRA, the person is no longer identified with PTSD, as a victim, or by any other label, and can look beyond self and family. New narratives of empowerment, resilience, and PTG begin to move the person to adopt a more altruistic perspective. In many cases, people in a state of PTG create something out of their trauma that is meaningful beyond their own personal healing and contributes to all of humanity.

We now return to the previous example of client Lita, to demonstrate how transformative roles emerge. After identifying how the trauma had been internalized, Lita wants to move off the Trauma Triangle. She chooses group members to play the roles she identified on the Triangle, her mother, father, and the victim—now her wounded child. Taking the role of appropriate authority, Lita goes to her wounded child and takes her off the Triangle to a safe place. In the role of the good-enough mother, she helps her younger self create a new narrative, telling her, "You are a beautiful child. I am so sorry your parents hurt you. They were wrong, and it was not your fault. I am here for you now and always will be. I will listen to you and take care of you." Lita role-reverses to take on the role of the wounded child, so she can experience being nurtured by a good-enough mother.

In the role of appropriate authority, Lita addresses her father, accurately labeling what happened: "There is nothing wrong with me or with my younger self. You are an alcoholic. And you acted cruelly and irresponsibly." Lita commands her father out of the circle of the drama, an action that begins to move the internalized perpetrator role out of her physiology. Continuing to create a new narrative, she addresses her mother: "You abandoned me, and that was wrong. You taught me to abandon myself. I will no longer do that. I could not stand up for myself then, but now I can." With the support of courage, Lita chooses a scarf to represent shame and addresses her parents: "This shame does not belong to me. It is yours. I know you were both mistreated as children and had no models for good parenting. I am giving this shame back to you. You can give it back to past generations, if you like." Some members of the group spontaneously take the role of past generations. Lita's parents take the scarf and pass it back to previous generations. Lita acknowledges that she has more work to do with her parents in the future.

As good-enough mother, she takes her wounded child in her arms, asking the prescriptive roles to surround them. The goddess (good-enough spirituality) sings, "How could anyone ever tell you, you were anything less than beautiful . . ." (Roderick, 2005), and everyone in the room joins her. Creativity (good-enough spirituality) invites Sandy and Molly (good-enough significant others) to help her lead the group in a dance with Lita and her sleeping-awakening Child in the center. Stepping into her ultimate authority role, Lita envisions taking the song and dance to the young students with whom she works.

CONCLUSION

The TSM is a psychodramatic, whole-person approach to working with people who have experienced trauma. The ultimate goal of TSM experiential psychotherapy is to not only treat trauma, but also lead to the development of the transformative roles of PTG. As we have seen, TSM psychodrama meets people where they are, honoring their experiences and working with the goals they have set for themselves, thus making it highly adaptable to diverse groups of people.

Through embodied experiences that follow the TSIRA clinical map, trauma survivors access their spontaneity and creativity by playing the prescriptive roles. With this internal support, they can face the trauma and take the actions needed to heal the past and develop new transformative roles for PTG. The TSIRA acts as a holding environment, containing them in their window of tolerance, so they can change their brains and nervous systems as they move through the three stages of the model. As their inner worlds change, trauma survivors become empowered to change their interpersonal *social atom*. The ultimate goal of TSM is for trauma survivors, and all people, to have full access to spontaneity and creativity, so they can step into the role of ultimate authority and cocreate a world that is beneficial to all of humanity (J. L. Moreno, 1947; Z. T. Moreno, 2012).

The Therapeutic Spiral Model and the Whole-Person Approach

TSM, like psychodrama, is a health model. Each person is viewed as a role player, and health is seen as the result of playing many roles and playing each one fully. Roles are embodied, affecting affect, behavior, and cognition. TSM prescribes the containment roles of BD and CD to anchor the client in the body and balance thinking and feeling. Although the TSIRA focuses on internalized roles, interpersonal roles are also addressed. People are recognized as having a *social atom*, which consists of the people and communities they find important.

TSM is *person-centered*, meaning there is genuine concern and respect for each person. Each subjective experience and story is unique and worthy of exploration. Each person's unique spirituality is honored as necessary for healing.

The theoretical basis and the methods of psychodrama focus on spontaneity training. *Spontaneity* is defined as the ability to have an adequate and appropriate response, which requires being in the present moment. TSM prescribes specific roles to increase spontaneity for trauma survivors to make needed changes in their lives. Having access to spontaneity and creativity affects every aspect of one's life.

QUALIFICATIONS AND TRAINING

Therapeutic Spiral International (TSI) provides a two-year certification program in trauma therapy using TSM. The program includes theory, practice, and supervision. There are eight required clinical courses, each lasting a minimum of three days and available as a stand-alone workshop. Courses contain immediately useful TSM clinical action intervention tools. The requirements for certification are at four levels of competency: trained auxiliary ego, assistant leader, team leader, and trainer. Each level requires practicum experience and supervision. A theory certification is available for those who only take the courses.

TSI training hours count toward certification by the Board of Examiners of Psychodrama, Sociometry and Group Psychotherapy, psychodrama requirements in Drama Therapy, and certification by the Society of Experiential Therapists. Psychodrama training supports TSM skill-building.

For certification in TSM, see https://therapeuticspiralmodel.com; for certification in psychodrama (by the American Board of Examiners of Psychodrama, Sociometry and Group Psychotherapy), see: https://www.psychodramacertification.org.

Evidence-Based Research

TSM is grounded in the research of neurobiology, experiential therapies, and psychodrama. Neurobiological research has shown that experiential methods are the treatment of choice for trauma prevention and repair; it also notes the efficacy of experiential therapies over cognitive behavioral therapy when working with trauma survivors. Moreover, psychodrama research has demonstrated significant improvements when applied to trauma survivors with addictions, dissociative identity disorder, and depression, as well as with sex offenders.

Quantitative research on TSM's CD has shown statistically significant decreases in dissociation, depression, anxiety, and general symptoms of PTSD, during a six-month follow-up after three individual therapy sessions. TSM's action protocol for a three-day weekend has produced increased self-esteem and connections for women who served in Afghanistan and Iraq.

Additional research is currently being conducted in Taiwan, Egypt, and the United States.

DIVERSITY/POPULATIONS

TSM has been used in more than 40 countries with trainers in Australia, Indonesia, Canada, China, Egypt, England, Germany, South Africa, Taiwan, and the United States. TSM'S Diploma Program in Egypt was approved by the Egyptian Group Therapy Association in 2013. TSM has been the foundational training for the first mental health centers at Hua Qiao and Nanjing Universities in China. Indeed, TSM has had a profound effect in China, where PTSD had not been recognized and symptoms of trauma were attributed to depression and lack of motivation.

Welcoming all people is in the tradition of psychodrama, with its goal to heal all of humankind. TSM groups explore commonalities and differences to establish safety before moving into trauma work. Because both psychodrama and TSM are known internationally, groups often reflect diverse ethnicities and races. Practitioners work with sensitivity to adapt the model appropriately. For example, a common practice in TSM groups is to create a circle of safety, with participants naming a strength they bring to the group. In China, where speaking highly of one's self goes against cultural norms, the circle of safety is created by group members naming a strength that they see in each participant.

Separate TSM men's and women's groups, and mixed-gender groups, are available. Those who identify as gender-fluid are always welcome. In TSM, all individuals are honored as unique human beings with their own history and experience.

TSM FOR PTSD IN A CLINICAL SETTING

When clients have experienced and understood the roles of the three stages of the TSIRA, they have acquired lifetime tools with which to work. There is a growing body of literature to support TSM's effectiveness with clients in ongoing groups, workshops, and couple and individual sessions. TSIRA charts and related articles are available online at https://therapeuticspiralmodel.com.

ACKNOWLEDGMENTS

The author wishes to thank Kate Hudgins and Francesca Toscani for their teachings and support in writing this chapter, and Dawn Blunk for her helpful editing.

REFERENCES

Badenoch, B. (2008). *Being a brain-wise therapist: A practical guide to interpersonal neurobiology*. New York: W. W. Norton.

Baim, C. (2013). Footsteps on the Moon: Using Therapeutic Spiral Model Concepts with Offenders who have Unresolved Trauma. In K. Hudgins & F. Toscani, *Healing world trauma with the therapeutic spiral model: Stories from the front-lines* (pp. 317–32). London, UK: Jessica Kingsley.

Burden, K., & Ciotola, L. (2002). The body double: An advanced clinical action intervention module in the therapeutic spiral model to treat trauma. Retrieved from www.vsjournals.de/pdf/body-offener-beitrag-032007.pdf.

Calhoun, L. G., & Tedeschi, R. G. (eds.). (2014). *Handbook of posttraumatic growth: Research and practice* (2nd ed). Mahwah, NJ: Lawrence Erlbaum Associates.

Carnabucci, K., & Ciotola, L. (2013). *Healing eating disorders with psychodrama and other action methods: Beyond the silence and the fury*. London: Jessica Kingsley.

Cozolino, L. J. (2002). *The neuroscience of psychotherapy: Building and rebuilding the human brain*. New York: W. W. Norton.

Cozolino, L. J. (2014). *The neuroscience of human relationships* (2nd ed). New York: W. W. Norton.

Cozolino, L. J. (2016). *Why therapy works: Using our minds to change our brains*. New York: W. W. Norton.

Gendlin, E. T. (1957). A descriptive introduction to experiencing. *Counseling Center Discussion Papers*, *3*(25). Chicago: University of Chicago (Special Collections: Archival Monographs) (8 pp.). Retrieved from http://www.focusing.org/gendlin/gol_primary_bibliography.htm.

Giacomucci, S. (2019). The trauma survivor's inner role atom: A clinical map for posttraumatic growth. *Journal of Psychodrama, Sociometry, and Group Psychotherapy*, *66*. In press.

Greenberg, L. S. (2013). Anchoring the Therapeutic Spiral Model into research on experiential psychotherapies. In K. Hudgins & F. Toscani (eds.), *Healing world trauma with the Therapeutic Spiral Model: Stories from the front lines* (pp. 132–48). London: Jessica Kingsley.

Greenberg, L. S., Watson, J. C., & Lietaer, G. (1998). *Handbook of experiential psychotherapy*. New York: Guilford Press.

Hudgins, M. K. (2001). *Experiential psychotherapy to treat trauma: The Therapeutic Spiral Model*. New York: Springer.

Hudgins, M. K. (2007). Clinical foundations of the Therapeutic Spiral Model: Theoretical orientations and principles of change. In C. Baim, J. Burmeister, & M. Maciel (eds.), *Psychodrama: Advances in theory and practice* (pp. 175–88). London: Routledge.

Hudgins, M. K. (2015). Spiral healing: A thread of energy and connection across cultures. In S. L. Brooke & C. E. Myers (eds.), *Therapists creating a cultural tapestry: Using the creative therapies across cultures* (pp. 260–81). Springfield, IL: Charles C Thomas.

Hudgins, M. K. (2017). PTSD unites the world: Prevention, intervention, and training in the Therapeutic Spiral Model. In C. E. Stout & G. Want (eds.), *Why global health matters: Guidebook for innovation and inspiration*. CreateSpace Independent Publishing Platform.

Hudgins, M. K., & Drucker, K. (1998). The Containing Double as part of the Therapeutic Spiral Model for treating trauma survivors. *International Journal of Action Methods*, *51*(2), 63–74.

Hudgins, M. K., & Kiesler, D. J. (1987). Individual experiential psychotherapy: An initial validation study of the intervention module of psychodramatic doubling. *Psychotherapy*, *24*, 245–55.

Hudgins, M. K., & Toscani, M. F. (eds.). (2013). *Healing world trauma with the Therapeutic Spiral Model: Stories from the front lines*. London: Jessica Kingsley.

Hudgins, M. K., Culbertson, R., & Hug, E. (2009). *Action against trauma: A trainer's manual for community leaders following traumatic stress*. Charlottesville: University of Virginia, Foundation for the Humanities, Institute on Violence and Culture. Retrieved from www.lulu.com/action-against-trauma-a-trainers-manual/6009176.

Hudgins, M. K., Drucker, K., & Metcalf, K. (2000). The containing double: A clinically effective psychodrama intervention for PTSD. *British Journal of Psychodrama and Sociodrama*, *15*(1), 58–77.

Hug, E. (2013). A neuroscience perspective on trauma and action methods. In K. Hudgins & F. Toscani (eds.), *Healing world trauma with the Therapeutic Spiral Model* (pp. 111–31). London: Jessica Kingsley.

Kellermann, P. F., & Hudgins, K. (2001). *Psychodrama with trauma survivors: Acting out your pain*. London: Jessica Kingsley.

McVea, C., & Gow, K. (2006). Healing a mother's emotional pain: Protagonist and director recall of a therapeutic spiral model session. *Journal of Psychodrama, Group Psychotherapy, and Sociometry*, *59*(1), 3–22.

Moreno, J. L. (1947). *The theater of spontaneity*. Beacon, NY: Beacon House.

Moreno, J. L. (1953). *Who shall survive? Foundations of sociometry, group psychotherapy, and sociodrama*. Beacon, NY: Beacon House.

Moreno, Z. T. (2012). *To dream again: A memoir*. Catskill, NY: Mental Health Resources.

Moreno, Z. T, Blomkvist, L. D., & Rützel, E. (2000). *Psychodrama, surplus reality, and the art of healing*. London: Routledge.

Moreno, Z. T., Horvatin, T., & Schreiber, E. (2006). *The quintessential Zerka: Writings by Zerka Toeman Moreno on psychodrama, sociometry, and group psychotherapy*. London: Routledge.

Panksepp, J. (1998). *Affective neuroscience: The foundations of human and animal emotions*. New York: Oxford University Press.

Perls, F. S., Hefferline, R. F., & Goodman, P. (1951). *Gestalt therapy*. New York: Julian Press.

Perry, R., Saby, K., Wenos, R., Hudgins, K., & Baller, M. (2016). Psychodrama intervention for female service members using the Therapeutic Spiral Model. *Journal of Psychodrama, Sociometry, and Group Psychotherapy*, *64*(1), 11–23.

Rezacian, M. P., Mazumdar, D. P. S., & Sen, A. K. (1997). The effectiveness of psychodrama in changing the attitudes among depressed patients. *Journal of Personality and Clinical Studies*, *13*, 19–23.

Roderick, L. (2005). *How could anyone*. Saskatoon, Canada: Turtle Island Records. Retrieved from www.Libbyroderick.com.

Siegel, D. (2007). *The mindful brain: Reflection and attunement in the cultivation of well-being*. New York: W. W. Norton.

Siegel, D. (2010). *The mindful therapist: A clinician's guide to midnight and neural integration*. New York: W. W. Norton.

Siegel, D. (2012). Developing mind: How relationships and the brain interact to shape who we are. New York: Guilford Press.

Stadler, C., Wieser, M., & Kirk, K. (eds.). (2016). Psychodrama: Empirical research and science 2. Psychodrama. Empirische Forschung und Wissenschaft 2 (Zeitschrift für Psychodrama und Soziometrie ed. Vol. 15, 1 supplement). Wiesbaden, Germany: Springer VS. Retrieved from http://link.springer.com/journal/11620/15/1/suppl/page/1; http://www.springer.com/de/book/9783658130145.

Toscani, M. F., & Hudgins, M. K. (1995). *The trauma survivor's intrapsychic role atom*. Workshop Handout. Madison, WI: Center for Experiential Learning.

Wieser, M. (2011). Studies on treatment effects of psychodrama psychotherapy. In C. M. D. Sales, G. Moita, & J. Frommer (eds.), *Methodological diversity in psychotherapy and counselling research: Qualitative-quantitative approach.* 1st International Summer School for Psychotherapy and Counseling Research: Proceedings (pp. 37–40, 111–24). Lisbon, Portugal: Universidade Autónoma de Lisboa. Retrieved from https://www.researchgate.net/publication/215867545_Studies_on_Treatment_Effects_of_Psychodrama_Psychotherapy.

Chapter Eight

Time-Focused Psychotherapy

Time Perspective Therapy

Rosemary Sword

In October 2008, my late husband, Richard Sword, and I attended the Hawaii Psychological Association's annual conference in Honolulu, where world-renowned researcher and educator Philip Zimbardo unveiled his fascinating and then-new book *The Time Paradox* (Zimbardo & Boyd, 2008). In his speech, Zimbardo detailed his Temporal Theory, whereby he divided time as we know it—the past, present, and future—into subsets of positive and negative experiences, that is, past positive and past negative. During the presentation, Rick and I realized that aspects of Zimbardo's concept of "time perspective" were similar to the way we helped our clients—the majority of whom were war veterans—suffering from posttraumatic stress disorder (PTSD). When one of the attendees asked Zimbardo if he had ever applied his Temporal Theory, Zimbardo replied that, as an academic researcher and psychologist, it was his job to indicate areas of concern; it was up to clinicians to develop solutions.

At the close of the event, Rick and I introduced ourselves to Zimbardo and discussed the possibility of adapting his time perspective therapy (TPT) for PTSD application. We explained that our focus with our clients had been accepting and honoring the past, seeking enjoyment in the present, and planning for the future. Now, Zimbardo had given us a language and an outline with which to work. Expressing interest in our idea, he asked us to stay in touch with him. This brief but significant encounter was the genesis of a professional relationship that would quickly lead to the development and implementation of what would become TPT.

TPT has a significantly different focus on the management of posttraumatic stress from that of previous models. Instead of replaying the trauma multiple times, TPT focuses on remembering the *positive* things of one's past rather than only the negatives, and then working in the present to create a brighter tomorrow. While TPT does not discount or gloss over traumatic memories (we clearly show respect for the origin of the trauma), we specifically avoid the trap of getting stuck in the traumatic negative past, which may increase its horrific effects via reliving it.

In TPT, we move forward, rather than continually looking backward. We learn from the past and recall the client's wonderful memories—some good times that happened at about the time of the traumatic event—on which we can build. This helps us overcome the negative events of the past and motivates us toward a brighter future.

This simple concept is reflected in the ordinary language that time perspective therapists use. Most people suffering from PTSD have already been labeled as anxious, depressed, or even "mentally ill." When they hear and identify with these words, they may conclude that the possibility of ever emerging from such a state is unattainable. We prefer to reframe their "illness" as a *mental injury*, recasting their depression and anxiety as a "negative past" experience that they can replace with a "positive present," a "brighter future," and, ultimately, a balanced time perspective. This approach may seem overly simplistic, especially to those trained in psychotherapy. But to PTSD survivors, the idea of having a forward-leaning framework in which to begin to understand and work with a therapist on their issues comes as an enormous relief and also a welcome ray of light in their previous darkness.

THE IMPORTANCE OF TIME PERSPECTIVES

We are all familiar with the three main time zones: the past, the present, and the future. In TPT, these time zones are divided into subsets: *past positive* and *past negative*, *present hedonism* and *present fatalism*, and *future positive* and *future negative*. When one of these time perspectives is too heavily weighted, we can lose out on what's really happening now and/or lose sight of what could be happening in our future, causing us to be unsteady, or unbalanced, or temporally biased.

Being out of balance in this way also shades the way we think by negatively impacting our daily decision-making process. For instance, if you are stuck in a past negative experience, you might think that from now on, everything that happens to you will be negative; so why would you even bother planning for your future, since it's just going to continue to be the same old bad stuff? Or, if you are an extreme present hedonist intent on spiking your adrenal glands, then you might engage in risky behaviors that unintentionally endanger yourself or others, because you are living in the moment and not thinking about future consequences of today's actions. If you are out of balance in your future time perspective, constantly thinking and worrying about all the things you have to do, you might forget or miss out on the everyday, wonderful things happening in your life and the lives of your loved ones in the here and now.

SIX MAIN TIME PERSPECTIVES IN TPT

The six main time perspectives in TPT are as follows:

1. *Past positive* people focus on the good things that have happened.
2. *Past negative* people focus on all the things that went wrong in the past.
3. *Present hedonistic* people live in the moment, seeking pleasure, novelty, and sensation, and avoiding pain. (However, since the development of TPT, we've noted that the ideal time perspective includes *moderate* present hedonism. It includes mindfulness of the present moment, sensory awareness, and mutuality in relationship.)
4. *Present fatalistic* people feel that planning for future decisions are not necessary, because predetermined fate plays the guiding role in one's life.
5. *Future positive* people plan for the future and trust that their decision will work out.
6. *Future negative* people feel that the future is fatalistic or apocalyptic, or have no future-orientation at all.

There is an additional subset of the future time-oriented people that can be called *transcendental future-oriented*. These people believe that, by leading a "good" life while on Earth, they will be rewarded in the afterlife. As a significant percentage of our clients do not believe in an afterlife, the transcendental future-orientation is not used in our version of TPT, but it could, of course, be included in treatment with specific clients.

The signature time perspective profile of an individual with PTSD is as follows: low past positive, high past negative; low (or high, depending on whether one is using this time perspective as a form of escape from reality) present hedonism, high present fatalism; and low or negative future orientation. In a nutshell, the goal in TPT is to balance negative time perspectives with positive ones. In other words, for people with PTSD, the idea is to boost past positive memories to help curb past negatives, introduce and practice selected present hedonism to offset present fatalism, and focus on building a brighter future to help reinforce hope, as opposed to thoughts of a negative future.

THREE MAIN TIME PERSPECTIVE BIASES

Past Bias

Good and bad things happen to everyone. But some of us view the world through rose-colored glasses (past positive), whereas others see the world through a darker lens (past negative). We have found that people who primarily focus on the past value the old more than the new; the familiar over the novel; and the cautious, conservative approach over the daring, more liberal, or risky one.

Present Bias

People who live in the present are far less—or not at all—influenced by either past experiences or future considerations. They focus on the immediate present—what's happening *now* (present hedonism). Most decisions are based on the immediate stimulus situation: internal hormonal signals, feelings, smells, sounds, the attractive qualities of the object of desire, and what others are urging them to do. Present-biased people who are influenced by past negative experiences are likely to feel stuck in the mire of the past *now* (present fatalism).

Future Bias

No one is born thinking about how to plan for the future. A number of conditions—including living in a temperate zone (where it is necessary to anticipate seasonal change), living in a stable family or stable economic/political society (where people learn to trust promises made to them), and becoming educated—can create future positive-oriented people. In general, future-oriented people do very well in life. They are less aggressive, are less depressed, have more energy, take care of their health, have good impulse control, and have more self-esteem. But those who are stuck in the past, locked into negative memories, and feeling fatalistic about the present, may have lost the ability even to conceive of a hopeful future (future negative).

TPT AND THE WHOLE-PERSON APPROACH

TPT addresses the whole-person approach, as it is a humanistic, client-centered, collaborative style of therapy that promotes the healing of the PTSD survivor through greater self-awareness, self-care, and social integration. As mentioned earlier, in TPT, posttraumatic stress is considered a mental *injury*, rather than a disorder or an illness. Like falling out of a tree and breaking your arm, when you suffer from PTSD, you can be fine one moment, and then you aren't. Similarly, when you suffer from an illness, you may be incurable; but when you have been injured, there is the possibility of recovery. TPT holds hope for the future, as well as continued growth throughout life. Its simplicity allows it to be easily grasped by clients, as evidenced in our work with veterans: As a result of TPT, they have been able to see themselves as cocoaches in their own therapy.

TPT begins by respecting the trauma for what it can teach us rather than dwelling on how it harmed us. It understands that we each have a unique time-perspective narrative based on our personal experiences, and this perspective is the lens through which we view our lives. But our experiences do not define us. They do not need to lock us into a particular way of seeing the world and our place in it—particularly when that way of seeing things is currently destructive to ourselves and those we love.

No matter what our experiences have been, the realization that we always have the choice to change how we view the times of our lives is essential. During the course of TPT, PTSD survivors move away from their traumatic past, pessimistic present, and negative thoughts of the future. Instead, they journey toward a *balanced time perspective* in which it once again seems possible to live a full and promising life in the present—learning to make time for what matters most: family, friends, fun, nature, hobbies, and constructive work.

QUALIFICATIONS AND TRAINING

My husband Rick was fond of saying, "We are going to take TPT out of the ivory tower and place it squarely in the hands of the people." Following through with Rick's idea, we have determined that individuals with an undergraduate degree in psychology can practice TPT as they would cognitive behavioral therapy (CBT). As an aside, in presentations and workshops, we found that students and laypeople absorbed TPT concepts as quickly as, and in some instances faster than, those with multiple degrees. Rick thought that it was because they were not weighed down by years of accumulated knowledge.

Although TPT was developed as a treatment for PTSD, it has proved effective for a wide range of uses (see "Diversity/Populations" later in this chapter). Aspects of TPT, for example, refocusing from past negatives to past positives and making plans for a brighter future positive, are practical for a variety of occupations aside from those in mental health, namely, medical practitioners, physical or massage therapists, alternative medicine practitioners, and school or university counselors.

The Time Cure Therapist Guidebook (Zimbardo, Sword, & Sword, 2014) was created for therapists and those seeking self-help interested in the step-by-step TPT process. *The Guidebook* is the template for TPT training. Due to the simplicity of TPT, which complements an already established practice or can be the main therapy in a new practice, additional training is unnecessary.

EVIDENCE-BASED RESEARCH

After meeting with Zimbardo in late 2008, Rick and I developed and commenced using TPT at our clinic on Maui with our clients, most of whom suffered from PTSD. We contacted Zimbardo soon thereafter to share our encouraging results. In June 2009, Zimbardo dispatched San Francisco-based researchers Sarah Brunskill and Anthony Ferreras to Maui for two weeks to conduct research on the effectiveness of TPT with regard to a test group of seasoned war veterans with severe PTSD. Baseline data had been established at the beginning of therapy by administering a battery of psychological tests: the Burns Depression Checklist, the Burns Anxiety Inventory, the Posttrauma Checklist for military, and, later, the Zimbardo Time Perspective Inventory (ZTPI).

As background related to the significance of the percentage gains experienced by the TPT participants, a 30% improvement is typically considered significant in psychological research. Usually, there is about a 20% improvement due just to the *placebo effect*, which is the subliminal expectation of getting well, even if there is no medical basis for it—that is, 20% of people will get better, regardless of whether they got the "real" treatment or merely believe that they did (Kapchuck, 2012). A similar term is the *halo effect*, which refers to the idea that a person's specific personality traits influence judgments by others about that person's global traits (Cherry & Fogoros, 2018).

In the TPT study, we were able to document—to a very high level of scientific confidence—that the veterans found improvements notably greater than either the placebo or the halo effect could account for. On average, positive treatment effects were found after only six to eight therapy sessions. These were encouraging results.

In the six-month period from January to June 2009, levels of depression improved 89%, levels of anxiety improved 70%, and levels of trauma improved 52%. The changes in depression and anxiety could only be accounted for by chance in less than one out of one thousand times. The changes in levels of trauma could only be accounted for by chance in fewer than one out of one hundred times. Clearly, TPT helped these veterans attain better scores on clinical assessments in comparison to their pretherapy test levels. It also proved consistent with the researchers' direct clinical observations of these veteran clients' behavior, as well as the qualitative assessment of them by their time perspective therapists and their own self-reports.

All 32 veterans were retested in June 2010. The improvements had endured, with slight improvements during the one-year period from June 2009 to June 2010. This is an important finding: The significant improvement in symptoms demonstrated in the first phase of the study was maintained, and almost two-thirds of the cases even improved during a one-year period.

In the June 2011 retest, two veterans were removed from the study, as they had relocated. But, of the remaining 30 veterans, their significant improvement in symptoms endured during a two-year period. Through follow-up interviews, the researchers discovered that a slight dip in trauma improvement from June 2010 to June 2011 was due to situational events that affect us all at some point in our lives, for example, health issues or death of a loved one; however, despite these normal life problems, the veterans continued to experience relief from trauma symptoms.

With each retest, the improvement in symptoms endured (Stolarski, Fieulaine, & van Beek, 2015). Overall, 87% of clients reported decreased trauma and PTSD symptoms, with an astonishing 100% decrease in their depression rating. This indicates that TPT is not a temporary fix; gains can be retained and even improved upon. In addition, during this four-year period, not a single veteran-client attempted suicide—in dramatic contrast to the high percentage of nontreated veterans who attempted or committed suicide during that same time frame. There are, moreover, no known risks in the implementation of TPT.

DIVERSITY/POPULATIONS

As TPT was originally developed to help those suffering from PTSD, it is, as one might expect, also efficacious in the treatment of depression, anxiety, and/or stress. It has proven effective in individual, couples, and family counseling for a variety of social problems. TPT works cross-culturally and cross-generationally, as evidenced in the research study mentioned earlier, as well as in our work with civilian clients. Moreover, TPT can be an effective method to reduce PTSD nightmares, which typically repeat traumas reflecting the negative past. At the start of the study, veteran participants ranged in age from the mid-20s (Middle East wars) to the mid-80s (World War II). Our practice is in Hawaii, which is arguably the most culturally diverse state, with Caucasians making up approximately 25% of the population. Hence, the study participants, as well as our other clients, are ethnically diverse. We should also mention that, while TPT has been used with children and teenagers with some success, we found that they had difficulty grasping a far-future orientation, due to an underdeveloped perspective on the future.

TPT FOR PTSD IN A CLINICAL SETTING

We are happy to share our method of conducting TPT in a clinical setting; here it is outlined in six sessions.

Session 1

Clients are given an overview of what will occur in this and the following five sessions. *(Note: Clients may want to discuss their trauma in detail. We suggest you ask them to share an abbreviated version, while assuring them that you will cover their trauma in detail during a later session; however, if your clients insist on reviewing their trauma in session 1, be flexible. If their disclosure causes you to proceed out of sequence, you can easily resume in subsequent sessions.)* In this session, introduce your clients to Zimbardo's Temporal Theory, the ZTPI, and TPT as part of their new educational orientation.

1. PTSD: Start by explaining that PTSD consists of three components: a) trauma, which leaves a person feeling b) depressed and c) anxious. Mention you will administer psychological tests in the following session to determine whether your client suffers from PTSD and, if so, to what degree—a little or a lot.
2. Zimbardo's Temporal Theory: Developed by Philip Zimbardo more than three decades ago, Temporal Theory divides the three known time zones—past, present, and future—into subcategories:

   - past negative—focusing on what went wrong in the past.
   - past positive—focusing on the good things that happened.
   - present hedonism—living in the moment; seeking pleasure, novelty, and sensation; and avoiding pain. People in this category may have an addictive personality. (The ideal present time perspective is *selected present hedonism*: a focus on a moderate amount of pleasure and sensation seeking, frequently as a reward for one's accomplishments. It also includes switching focus from one's self to others, that is, being with and/or helping others in some way; this is encouraged as an increased sense of belonging and feeling like one is part of a community, and can help reduce negative thoughts and actions.)
   - present fatalism—feeling that decisions are moot because predetermined fate plays the guiding role in life. In the extreme, people in this category believe that nothing good will ever happen.
   - future negativism (fatalistic or no future)—being convinced that everything will be bad or will not turn out well.

- future positivism—planning for the future and trusting that decisions made will work out.

3. Zimbardo Time Perspective Inventory (ZTPI): This is the key tool used in TPT to determine clients' time perspective profiles. Developed by Phil Zimbardo and John Boyd (*The Time Paradox*, 2008), the ZTPI is a 56-statement psychological test that gives the therapist and the client an idea of their different time perspective scores. *A separate "transcendental" inventory is also available to determine the level of belief the client has in an afterlife; however, this inventory is not used in TPT.*

Ryan Howell developed the 15-item ZTPI short form provided in session 2. The 56-statement ZTPI, or the ZTPI short form, as well as the three tests—or similar ones—mentioned earlier are to be administered in the next session.

Conclude the session by suggesting that clients view the timeperspective-therapy.org website to familiarize themselves with the process, as well as the 20-minute *The River of Time* video on YouTube, which was especially created to assist clients in the TPT process. Your clients' homework is to view *The River of Time* once a day until the next session. Explain that the video contains a breathing technique that is an important part of their TPT; they are to learn and practice it. *(Note: If you have practiced a specific breathing technique during previous therapy with your clients, there is no need to change to the suggested TPT technique.)* If you have time, take your clients to the aforementioned websites to familiarize them in advance, in your presence.

Session 2

Confirm to the best of your ability that your clients actually suffer from PTSD. This is accomplished by administering the ZTPI, as well as trauma, anxiety, and depression tests. We used the Posttrauma Checklist—Civilian, if working with civilian clients, or the Posttrauma Checklist—Military, if working with a military service personnel or veteran clients, as well as the Burns Anxiety Inventory and the Burns Depression Checklist. We have found it most helpful to use paper copies of the ZTPI (see "Additional Resources"). This allows you to keep the copy in your clients' files for future reference. The 15-statement ZTPI short form is included here to give you an idea of what these inventories are like; it also enables you to take the test yourself. During this session, you will do the following:

1. Explain test scoring since psychological tests may score differently; be sure to explain how each test is scaled. For example, some tests are

scaled 1 to 5, with 1 = "not at all" (no symptoms), 2 = "a little bit" (minimal symptoms), 3 = "moderately" (moderate symptoms), 4 = "quite a bit" (severe symptoms), and 5 = "extremely" (extreme trauma symptoms). ZTPI scales are as follows: 1 = very untrue, 2 = untrue, 3 = neutral, 4 = true, 5 = very true—about ME (the client).

2. Administer psychological tests and the ZTPI. Ask your clients each item on the trauma, depression, and anxiety tests, and total the scores. When taking the ZTPI, your clients may get stuck in thoughts or feelings; note the areas you or your clients may wish to explore later and continue with the ZTPI until it is complete. If your clients have difficulty deciding on an answer, then mark 3 (neutral) and move on to the next item. If your clients want to take the psychological tests and the ZTPI on their own, allow them ample time (perhaps the entire session) to finish the tests.
3. Explain that you will review the results in the next session. If you have additional time in session 2, consider exploring one or more of the areas of concern you marked earlier in the ZTPI.
4. Prior to session 3, review your clients' trauma, depression, and anxiety scores to determine the depth of their PTSD. If you have administered the ZTPI in paper form, go to the www.thetimeparadox.com website and input your clients' responses to each ZTPI statement. Print up your clients' scores, plot the scores on the graph (see session 3), and staple the results to the front of your clients' hard copies of the ZTPI, noting which scores are highest and lowest. The graph is a visual blueprint for you to share with your clients; it shows what time perspectives you and your clients will work toward to gain an ideal time perspective.

Your clients' scores will likely be as follows: low past positive, high past negative, low present hedonism, and low future. Explain how people suffering from PTSD are generally normal people who have been through a trauma that changes almost every aspect of their lives. Having difficulty with situations that prior to the trauma would have been handled with ease is common in PTSD sufferers. The key is *equal and opposite action for reaction*—in other words, to gain mental well-being, counteract negativity with positivity. Focus will be on boosting past positive memories to curb past negatives, introducing selected present hedonism to offset present fatalism, and making plans for a brighter future to replace future negative thoughts.

ZTPI SHORT FORM

Read each item and, as honestly as you can, answer the question, "How characteristic or true is this of me?" Please answer all the following questions. (Clinician: Use the scale below.)

From 1 (very untrue) to 5 (very true)

1. I think about the bad things that have happened to me in the past.
2. Painful past experiences keep being replayed in my mind.
3. It's hard for me to forget unpleasant images of my youth.
4. Familiar childhood sights, sounds, and smells often bring back a flood of wonderful memories.
5. Happy memories of good times spring readily to mind.
6. I enjoy stories about how things used to be in the "good old times."
7. Life today is too complicated; I would prefer the simpler life of the past.
8. Since whatever will be will be, it doesn't really matter what I do.
9. Often luck pays off better than hard work.
10. I make decisions on the spur of the moment.
11. Taking risks keeps my life from becoming boring.
12. It is important to put excitement in my life.
13. When I want to achieve something, I set goals and consider specific means for reaching those goals.
14. Meeting tomorrow's deadlines and doing other necessary work comes before tonight's play.
15. I complete projects on time by making steady progress.

Scale: past negative: 1, 2, 3; past positive: 4, 5, 6; present fatalism: 7, 8, 9; present hedonism: 10, 11, 12; future: 13, 14, 15.

Plot the scores on the Time Perspective Profile Score Sheet (see figure 8.1). Disregard the transcendental future score, which is a separate test and not used in TPT.

Session 3: The Past

1. Review: Begin by lightly touching upon your clients' compliance with practicing the breathing technique on a daily basis. Ask if they have had the opportunity to employ it during times of stress and, if so, if they found it helpful. If not, discuss why. Reiterate the importance of continued practice to make it part of their daily routine.
2. Test results: Share your clients' psychological test results (re: trauma, depression, and anxiety). Explain their scores (minimal to no, minimal, moderate, severe, or extreme). If their scores are severe to ex-

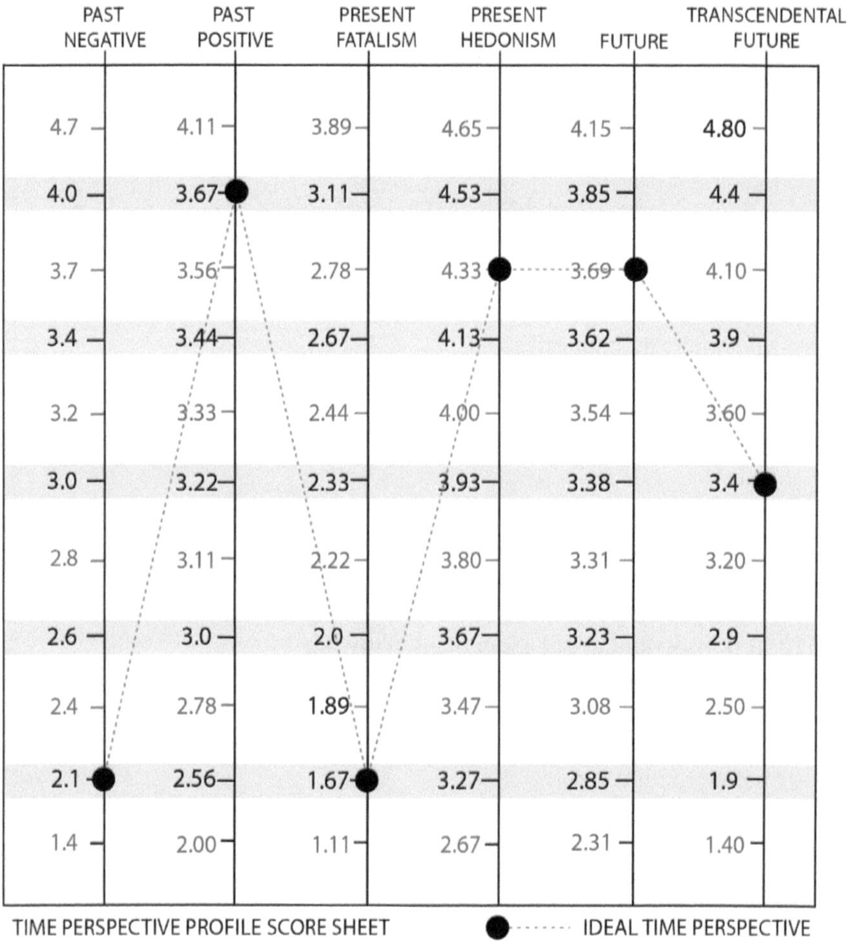

Figure 8.1. Time Perspective Profile Score Sheet. ***Rosemary K. M. Sword***

treme and this is upsetting to them, assuage their apprehension by telling them you will work together to improve their symptoms.

3. ZTPI: Show your clients theirTime Perspective Profile Score Sheet. PTSD sufferers usually have high past negative scores, because their trauma keeps them stuck in their traumatic past. Their second highest score is generally present fatalistic or present hedonistic.
4. High scores: Explain one or two of the highest scores. Certain high-score combinations—past negative/present fatalistic, past negative/present hedonistic, past negative/future (negative/fatalistic)—are the hallmarks of trauma, depression, and/or anxiety.

5. Low scores: Explain the one or two of the lowest scores. The low-score combinations of past positive/present hedonistic and past positive/future (positive) are also the hallmarks of trauma, depression, and/or anxiety.
6. Comparison: Compare and discuss your clients' scores with the suggested Ideal Time Perspective scores on the ZTPI graph (contact us at www.timeperspective.org for the graph in Word or .pdf).
7. Sharing: Ask your clients to share with you a few past positive memories. If they have difficulty remembering anything positive, explain that they do, indeed, have past positive memories, but these have been overshadowed by their past negatives, which negate positive recollections. If your clients have undergone severe trauma, it is best to ask them to recall past positives prior to the trauma. If they still cannot recall past positives, suggest that they imagine, if they *could* have had a past positive experience, what it would have been like. These two suggestions will likely lead them to remembering an actual past positive, followed by additional positive memories. Ask about their best buddies, best birthday, best gift they ever received, and so forth, to prime the pump of good thoughts.
8. Explain: Tell your clients that, whenever they have a past negative flashback or thought, they ought to replace it immediately with one of their past positive memories. Use specific individualized examples for your clients. For instance, if they were in a motor vehicle accident and have flashbacks while driving, ask them to recall a positive experience while driving, for instance, singing along to a favorite song on the radio, enjoying the anticipation of reaching their destination, or deciding which car they would like best to drive regardless of cost. If your clients cannot recall *any* positive experiences while driving, ask them to remember a time when they felt safe and comforted, and try to use this past positive memory when they experience a flashback.
9. Practice: Review replacing past negatives with past positives with your clients. If there is time remaining in the session, revisit one or more of the areas of concern you noted when your clients took the ZTPI.

Session 4: The Present

1. Review: Begin by checking your clients' progress in replacing past negatives with past positives. If they have been having trouble, ask them to explain exactly what happens at these times. If they find it impossible to replace a severe traumatic flashback with a positive past experience, spend time reviewing past positive memories until they can easily recall them. Then ask them to practice recalling past posi-

tives throughout the day so that when a past negative occurs they can more easily draw upon the past positive memory or memories. The plan is for these practices to become habitual and not limited to treatment sessions.

2. Selected present hedonism: You and your clients will employ *selected* present hedonism to offset extreme present hedonism or present fatalism. Prosocial behavior is an important aspect of TPT and is greatly encouraged; when one has PTSD, it is easy to forget about the things—and, perhaps more significantly, the people—that play key roles in our lives. It offsets the tendency toward self-imposed isolation (antisocial behavior) experienced by many suffering from PTSD. Ask your clients what they enjoy doing. If they do not do anything other than work and/or isolate at home, ask them what they enjoyed doing *prior* to their trauma. Then suggest that they take up that activity again. If they are unable to do so, for whatever reason—for example, an acquired disability—explore other feasible options.

   The following are some suggestions to initiate prosocial present hedonistic behavior:

   - Reconnect via telephone or e-messaging with a family member or friend with whom your client has not felt like speaking since the trauma.
   - Have a daily meal with family members or a friend instead of isolating in a room or at home.
   - Participate in community or social functions that used to be of interest.

3. Prosocial behavior: If appropriate, you may wish to discuss with your clients the possibility of bringing a family member or members into subsequent sessions to assist your clients in the therapeutic process. During the family session(s), briefly explain Temporal Theory and the TPT process so the family members understand what your clients are going through. On their own time, they might also take the ZTPI to become familiar with TPT terminology.
4. Revisit: If there is ample time remaining in the session, revisit one or more of the areas of concern you noted when your clients took the ZTPI initially.
5. Session conclusion: End the session on an upbeat note by reinforcing that you are working together in the TPT process to help your clients learn simple and doable ways to improve their lives in the present—more as teammates than as clients and therapist.

Session 5: The Future

1. Review: Begin by checking your clients' progress in doing the following:

   - Replacing past negatives with past positives.
   - Practicing their selected present hedonism/new prosocial behaviors. Discuss what they have been doing in these areas to improve their lives. If they are having difficulty, find out why and make appropriate suggestions (perhaps by reviewing session 4, number 5). Explain how good memories lead to past positives, which are processed in the present. While in the present, your clients can create hopes and dreams, and work toward a bright future positive.

2. Assist: Help your clients in making both short- and long-range plans for their brighter future. So that this is not an overwhelming task, start with their plans for the following day, followed by the week, the next two weeks, and so on. If they have difficulty with accomplishing daily activities due to lack of concentration and pace, suggest that they make a list of things they'd like to accomplish, for instance, organizing and paying bills, attending physician/therapist appointments, shopping or carrying out selected household chores, spending time with important people in their lives, and so forth. The list can be made and updated daily or weekly. Explain that there is no pass or fail but that the goal in this process is to accomplish one or two of the items on their list each day, thereby proving to themselves that they are capable of planning for their future and following through with their plans. Areas to cover are occupational, as well as social (family, friends, and acquaintances).
3. Revisit: If there is time remaining in the session, revisit one or more of the areas of concern you noted when your clients took the ZTPI.

Session 6: Balanced Time Perspectives Review

1. Review: Begin by checking your clients' progress. By this time, they should be practicing their breathing technique on a daily basis. They should also be able to replace all or most of their past negatives with past positives; however, if they are continuing to have difficulty, review session 4, number 1. Your clients should also be well on the way to practicing selected present hedonism and new prosocial behaviors. Discuss their progress. If they are having difficulty, talk about why and make appropriate suggestions. Review their future positive goals. Were they able to meet their short-term goals? If not, find out why.

2. Reinforce: Remind clients that, previously, their PTSD had kept them locked in their past negative trauma, but hopefully they have made good progress in reframing their past and are now equipped to plan for their brighter future positive while living in a more fulfilling present.
3. Revisit: If there were any areas of concern you noted when your clients took the ZTPI in session 2, now is the time to address them. At this point in the TPT process, your clients may see that these are old issues with which they have learned to deal through TPT. If an issue is more deep-seated (e.g., abuse of any type—drug or alcohol, physical, sexual, or mental), additional therapy may be necessary. Assure your clients that you will continue to work with them on these specific issues in future therapy.
4. Session conclusion: During this or a follow-up session, you may want to ask clients to take the ZTPI again. Scores may be reviewed and compared to their previous ZTPI scores as administered in session 2. You will know that your clients understand and are implementing TPT in their lives if their scores have improved.

BEING FLEXIBLE

Although we have used a logical progression in the development of each session, one of the beautiful things about TPT is the ability to move freely from one time perspective to another. We have found in our private clinical practice that some clients require additional time during one or more steps in the TPT process, or certain time perspectives may require immediate attention, superseding the suggested progression. The former usually occurs during session 1, at which time the clients' need to review past negative trauma(s) replaces the therapy process outlined earlier. As the clients' traumas are treated with great respect in TPT, you may have to spend two or more sessions reviewing their trauma and how it has affected their lives. If this is the case, please do so. But by the fourth session we suggest getting back on track with the TPT process as outlined previously. It is rare that immediate present or future needs supplant the suggested TPT process; when this has been the case with our clients, we have been able to leap from session 1 to session 5, number 2, and then back to sessions 2, 3, and 4, with a refresher session 5, concluding with session 6—with good results. Do feel free to improvise, as needed.

Remember: Having a balanced time perspective—high past positive, moderate selected present hedonism, including focus on random acts of kindness and helping others, and moderately high positive future with low past negative and low present fatalism—is the goal. This is the ideal time perspective combination for all of us to achieve.

REFERENCES

Cherry, K., & Fogoros, R. N. (2018, May 1). The halo effect and how it affects you. Retrieved from https://www.verywellmind.com/what-is-the-halo-effect-2795906.

Grant, A. M., & Berry, J. W. (2011). The necessity of others is the mother of invention: Intrinsic and prosocial motivations, perspective-taking, and creativity. *Academy of Management Journal, 54*(1), 73–96.

Kapchuck, T. (2012, April). Putting the placebo effect to work. Retrieved from https://www.health.harvard.edu/mind-and-mood/putting-the-placebo-effect-to-work.

Peterson, C. (2006). *A primer in positive psychology*. Oxford, UK: Oxford University Press.

Stolarski, M., Fieulaine, N., & van Beek, W. (eds.). *Time Perspective Theory; Review, research, and application.* New York: Springer.

Sword, R. M., Sword, R. K.M., & Brunskill, S. R. (2015). Time Perspective Therapy: Transforming Zimbardo's Temporal Theory into clinical practice. In M. Stolarski, N. Fieulaine, & W. van Beek (eds.), *Time Perspective Theory; Review, research, and application* (pp. 481–98). New York: Springer.

Sword, R. M., Sword, R. K. M., Brunskill, S. R., & Zimbardo, P. G. (2014). Time Perspective Therapy: A new time-based metaphor therapy for PTSD. *Journal of Loss and Trauma, 19*(3), 197–201. doi: 10.1080/15325024.2013.763632.

Zimbardo, P. G., & Boyd, J. (2008). *The Time Paradox: The new psychology of time that will change your life.* New York: Rider. Visit www.timeparadox.com to view the ZTPI long form, which can be taken online and scored automatically.

Zimbardo, P. G., Sword, R. K. M., & Sword, R. M. (2012). *The time cure: Overcoming PTSD with the new psychology of Time Perspective Therapy*. San Francisco, CA: Wiley.

Zimbardo, P. G., Sword, R. K. M., & Sword, R. M. (2014). *The time cure therapist guidebook*. San Francisco, CA: Wiley. Available at no charge from www.timeperspectivetherapy.org/comments/.

ADDITIONAL RESOURCES

The River of Time. Video. Retrievable from https://www.youtube.com/watch?v=r4ZX0XVAa2A .

Time Perspective Therapy. Contact us via the comment tab at www.timeperspectivetherapy.org for free pdfs of the 56-statement ZTPI and/or the short form, as well as the ZPTI graph and *The Time Cure Therapist Guidebook.*

III

Interventions for Communities

Chapter Nine

Israel Trauma and Resiliency Center—NATAL

Twenty Years of Coping with Invisible Wounds

Judith Yovel Recanati and
the NATAL Professional Team

When the State of Israel was established in 1948, after the Holocaust, it was immediately forced into a War of Independence, which took the lives of 1% of the population. Israel continues to exist in a condition of constant threats, recurrent wars, and ongoing terror attacks. In this ongoing traumatic reality, under the shadow of a massive collective trauma, NATAL (formerly known as the Israel Trauma Center for Victims of Terror and War) was established in 1998.

NATAL is an apolitical NGO that serves as a multidisciplinary therapeutic home for trauma casualties related to the Israel–Arab conflict. NATAL is governed by a comprehensive professional philosophy that addresses the various circles of traumatic impact. These include the following: the individual casualty and his/her family—through a unique Helpline, along with a traditional clinical staff; the community, via an outreach unit that works to prevent and reduce traumatic impact, promote resilience, and conduct emergency interventions; mental health professionals through NATAL's trauma-focused psychotherapy school; and Israeli society through the public relations and communications unit, which works to increase visibility, awareness, and the legitimacy of the discourse regarding war and terror-related trauma. More than 290,000 Israelis have been helped by NATAL. In this chapter, the professional activities and operating philosophy of the various units will be described and demonstrated via case studies showing best practices and interunit cooperation.

NATAL's unique model will be discussed in terms of the following: using a whole-person approach; maintaining an emphasis on continuity of care; and addressing various target populations, from the individual casualty with posttrauma and his/her relatives, through the community under threat, to society as a whole. We focus on the traumatic timeline: promoting resilience and increasing preparedness, before real-time intervention and treating post-traumatic casualties.

NATAL's model relates to trauma through the two prisms of personal individual trauma and the trauma of the collective ("national trauma"). Thus, we offer the possibility of considering trauma as a potential bridge to unite and promote understanding, acceptance, and opportunities for two societies, the Israeli and the Palestinian, entangled in the shackles of trauma and yearning for a peaceful resolution.

NATAL: ESTABLISHMENT AND TWO DECADES OF AN ACTIVE ROLE IN ISRAELI SOCIETY

In June 1998, a brief advertisement in an Israeli newspaper invited individuals who were struggling with the experiences of their military service or had survived terror attacks, to contact a new trauma center in Tel Aviv. The first request for help was received with excitement. Yossi Hadar, MD, cofounder and initiator of NATAL's concept and my partner in this endeavor, received the first client for an intake session. Unfortunately, the next day, Yossi Hadar was urgently admitted to the hospital and diagnosed with acute leukemia; he tragically passed away two weeks later, in July 1998. NATAL thus entered the world with this traumatic loss at its foundation, with its future about to be tested. My motivation for changing the course of my life and establishing this unique organization is presented here.

I was born in Tel-Aviv in the early 1950s, two years after the War of Independence (1948) and six years after the end of World War II. I spent my childhood in Tel-Aviv, against the background of the Sinai War (1956). As a teenager, I witnessed the Six-Day War (1967), after which there were terror attacks, killings, and tensions throughout Israel, followed by the War of Attrition. Immediately after my discharge from the Israel Defense Forces (IDF) in 1973, the Yom Kippur War broke out and left us, the first generation born after the establishment of the State, shocked, sad, and in pain. Ceremonies for Holocaust Remembrance Day and Memorial Day for fallen IDF soldiers, along with tragic events that preceded the establishment of the State of Israel, heightened my sense of identity and purpose, and were interwoven with great sadness for those who had given their lives for the continued existence of the Jewish State.

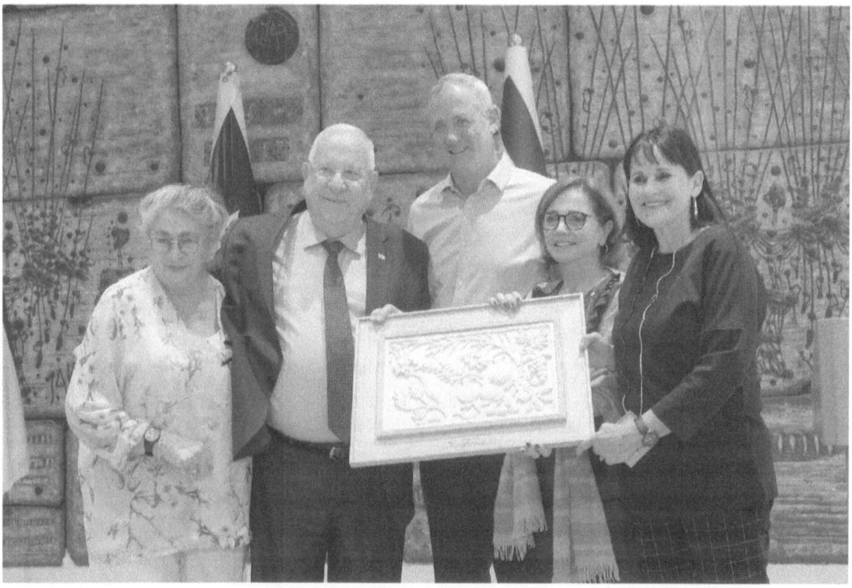

Figure 9.1. NATAL's 20 years of impact on Israeli society was commemorated at a special ceremony held at the residence of President Reuvin Rivlin in March 2018. In picture (right to left): NATAL executive director Orly Gal; NATAL founder and chairperson Judith Yovel Recanati; chairperson of the Public Advisory Committee, Lt. Gen. (res) Benny Gantz; President Reuvin Rivlin and his wife, Nechama Rivlin. *Aviv Hof/Judith Yovel Recanati*

When I was 35, my parents both died from severe illnesses. Their deaths affected me deeply, leading me to choose art therapy as my profession. I invested many years in studies at Lesley College in Boston, the School of Psychotherapy at Bar Ilan University, and courses and personal mentoring throughout my therapeutic work in various rehabilitation settings.

After Yossi Hadar's tragic death, NATAL became an integral part of my life. I understood that fate had intervened once again and introduced me to my life's mission: to ensure that NATAL achieved its goals. NATAL is an organization that grew from within Israeli society, for Israel, and for the emotional well-being and resilience of its citizens who suffer from posttraumatic stress following terror attacks or war.

From the beginning, NATAL's community teams have been, and remain, in contact with Jewish and non-Jewish Israelis, including Arab professionals, Jewish-Arab women's groups in mixed cities, and Arab schools.

Helpline: Telephone Interventions for Terror- and War-Related Trauma

NATAL's Helpline offers emotional support for citizens and army veterans who have been injured physically and/or psychologically in terror attacks and war, and individuals who have been emotionally affected by the security situation in Israel. This is a unique feature of NATAL, used as a model throughout the world.

A traumatic event (e.g., a terror attack) is like a stone thrown into the water, creating growing circles of casualties. The victims who were directly exposed are the inner circle. The second circle is comprised of the victims' close relatives, who care for their injured loved ones and experience feelings similar to theirs. The broader circles include neighbors, friends, distant relatives, and other citizens who experience a sense of threat and violation of personal safety on a daily basis (Tamir & Haimov, 2005). Analysis of the calls to NATAL's Helpline have consistently revealed that approximately 50% of the callers are direct victims, about 30% are family members of the victims, and an additional 20% experience distress related to the security situation, although they have not been directly or indirectly injured (Gelkopf, Haimov, & Lapid, 2015).

The stigma and the shame of mental illness remain top reasons why people choose to forgo care (Clement et al., 2015; Rüsch et al., 2006). It is sometimes hard to make the necessary connection between the traumatic event and one's present complicated mental state. Helplines offer a nonstigmatic service, while the anonymity and privacy make it easier to take this first step toward recovery. From the moment callers contact the Helpline, they are welcomed into a holding environment that is deliberately nonclinical. NATAL's Helpline is staffed by paraprofessional volunteers, who accompany callers with care and empathy, and constitute part of the community to which the victims belong. The callers' ability to make use of the community is an initial step toward renewing their connection with society (Herman, 1994). Additionally, paraprofessional volunteers were found to be most effective in crisis interventions (Lester & Rogers, 2012). NATAL's training course for Helpline volunteers, which is seven months long, includes weekly four-hour sessions and three additional months of group supervision. Once the volunteers begin working on regular shifts, they continue to have bimonthly supervision by professionals. Using volunteers instead of professionals brings a humanistic touch to this environment.

Options Offered by NATAL's Helpline

Onetime Intervention Model

The Onetime Intervention Model, by telephone or chat, aims to enable ventilation of feelings of distress, anxiety, and confusion, which undermine the sense of personal safety. Volunteers provide psychoeducational interventions by explaining the symptoms callers are experiencing and guiding them in improving their functioning. Most callers benefit from the intervention and are invited to call again whenever they need additional help. Psychoeducational interventions are associated with improved functioning and quality of life, decreased symptomatology, and positive outcomes for both the individuals with illness and their family members (Lukens & McFarlane, 2004). After a terror attack, people suffering from anxiety or stress may need immediate intervention; in this case, they are referred to the community outreach team for mobile unit initial intervention. If necessary, victims are offered long-term intervention via the Helpline or referral to NATAL's clinical unit. Our experience shows that primary intervention that provides ventilation, legitimacy, and psychoeducation is often an adequate response to victims' needs.

Ongoing Intervention Model

The Ongoing Intervention Model, by telephone or chat, was developed by NATAL based on Judith Herman's (1994) three stages of recovery from trauma. These include a) establishing a feeling of safety and stability for victims, followed by b) reconstructing the traumatic narrative, and then c) reconnecting the victims with people and meaningful activities. This model offers callers who need more than a onetime session an ongoing significant relationship. The Helpline volunteer calls once a week, on a designated day and at a designated time, and speaks with the client for 20 minutes. The intervention starts with building a therapeutic alliance, whose goal is to ease the loneliness that often characterizes trauma victims. The intervention aids in processing the traumatic event, while providing support during a difficult time and extending the range of interpretations and options through strengthening coping methods.

House Calls

The third option, house calls, is designed for trauma victims who feel a threat to their personal safety, which leads them to remain shut in their homes, socially isolated and with limited functioning. Using a structured program of house calls, NATAL's Helpline volunteers encourage, assist, and accompany the victims on their journey toward better functioning and gradual reinvolvement with life in the community.

NATAL offers flexibility and mobility between its various units. Many individuals who begin with a Helpline contact are later referred to the clinical unit for further treatment. The handover between the two units is attended by the same volunteer and the professional Helpline staff member. NATAL's Helpline and the clinical unit developed a unique protocol for preparing clients for clinical therapy, one that helps to evaluate clients' readiness for therapy, via a thorough examination of their exact needs, and provides scaffolding to increasing levels and continuity of care.

The benefits of NATAL's unique Helpline model are reflected in the following letter sent by one of our clients:

> After the attack I was so confused, afraid, and helpless that I didn't understand what was happening to me. I stopped eating, cried, didn't leave home, and couldn't sleep at night. Th phone calls with you helped calm me down and get organized. You helped me understand what was happening to me. You were the only ones [with whom] I could discuss my many difficulties. Thanks to your warm and caring approach, support, and patience, I was able to recuperate, and I now feel that I am on the road to recovery.

NATAL's Helpline serves as the main portal to the clinical unit. together with referrals from the Community Outreach Unit and its mobile unit work. Normally, the process begins in clinical meetings with social workers from the Helpline, who process calls and prepare for ongoing intervention via phone. Referrals for the clinical unit assess the traumatic event and the client's readiness and suitability for treatment. Therapeutic goals and preferred modalities of therapy are also evaluated at intake. A client's progress is evaluated semiannually by the therapists and unit director, as well as by self-assessment questionnaires filled out by the client. When additional psychopathology is suspected and a different diagnosis may be needed, the client is referred for psychiatric (re)evaluation. Thus, a large number of services are integrated into one coherent treatment model.

NATAL'S CLINICAL UNIT

NATAL's clinical unit offers therapy to Israeli civilians traumatized by terror and war, and to their supporting circles nationwide. The therapeutic conversation is based on a broad perspective of trauma and its grave ramifications. Intervention aims at reducing the client's suffering as expressed in symptoms and posttraumatic residues, which impact various strata of life. The approach emphasizes continuity of therapeutic processes through additional NATAL units, for example, community outreach.

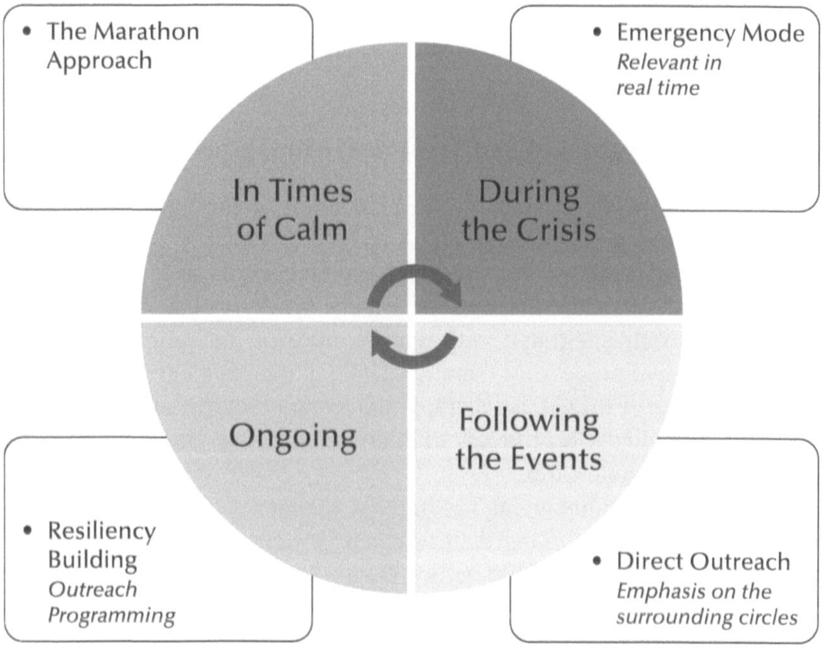

Figure 9.2. An example of how NATAL operates across the timeline of before, during, and after emergencies. ***Judith Yovel Recanati***

Guidelines for Intervention

The formation of a *safe place* for both clients and therapists serves as a key factor. It derives from the understanding that traumatized victims of terror and war have lost trust in both themselves and their environment. They perceive the world as a dangerous place in which they are liable to get hurt again at any moment. We aim to reestablish the experience of a safe place, one that radiates into to the world outside the clinic. This allows clients to gradually establish confidence in themselves and their capabilities.

The Young Veterans' Project makes a point of offering therapy as soon as possible after military service. The sooner treatment is provided, the more effective it is in preventing severe PTSD, reducing secondary damage among family and friends, and thereby reducing the need for disability claims.

The "whole-person" comprehensive approach is NATAL's flagship. For many clients, therapy programs combine at least two modalities (individual therapy, group therapy, spouse therapy, psychiatric monitoring, and a socio-rehabilitation club), integrating them with a base in a supportive and client-centered relationship. We do not treat them as patients, but as part of our community. We aim to not only restore balance to individuals, but also reintegrate them back into their communities. Given that Israel is a small country, everyone knows the soldiers, and the soldiers remain close to their families, so that healing for the soldiers requires healing for the entire community.

Therapeutic Approaches and Treatment Modalities

Forming a therapeutic alliance is the foundation of the process. It enables confidence building between the client and the therapist. It permits an open discussion about feelings, thoughts, and experiences, as well as the integration of several methods. Therapy is usually based on the principles of a dynamic approach integrated with one or more of the following: trauma-oriented cognitive processing therapy (CPT), eye movement desensitization and reprocessing (EMDR), art therapy, movement therapy, and "safe touch" therapy. Some clients receive an additional supporting framework through the Social Therapeutic Club.

NATAL's Psychohistorical Testimonial Center enables clients to give a video testimony documenting their traumatic events, thereby allowing them to present their narrative of life before, during, and after the event(s). It is up to the clients to decide what to do with their testimony; some choose to share it with family, and others to keep it private.

Structure and Working Processes

The following is an example of integrated treatment, which we call the story of family D.

The mother of family D was killed in a terror attack. Following the event, national security referred the father, the 14-year-old daughter, and the 13- and 8-year-old sons to NATAL. The children's functioning became chaotic, as they struggled to cope with the complex traumatic bereavement following their dominant mother's death. The father struggled to fulfill his role, with the additional tasks of running the home. Verbal and physical violence toward the children was described. The children were increasingly absent from school, and the daughter developed an eating disorder. NATAL decided on a tailor-made art therapy–oriented family program, with specific additional modalities for each member.

The father attended individual therapy and participated in the Social Therapeutic Club; the adolescent daughter attended individual therapy until she started mandatory military service at age 18, during which support continued via telephone conversations; the middle son was, likewise, in individual therapy, as well as biofeedback and safe touch therapy programs. Both boys were in psychiatric follow-up care. A Helpline volunteer supported the youngest son for three years, also modeling for the father. A female family therapist, who was filling the void caused by the mother's absence, maintained contact with the children's schoolteachers. The holistic integrative program and long-term extensive care succeeded in reducing the level of violence by improving the father's functioning and helped other family members continue to process their traumatic grief and achieve satisfactory levels of functioning in various life domains.

NATAL's therapeutic process is based on an extensive holistic view. It applies various integrative therapeutic modalities in a tailor-made fashion. Securing continuity of care is a key factor in determining the required duration of process for each individual. Sensitivity, empathy, and compassion accompany the clinical care process, allowing the client a sense of safety. This enables appropriate processing and restoration of self-confidence, and facilitates awareness, insight, and hope for change and growth. Outcomes indicate that NATAL's clinical practice indeed enables change and leads to improvement in life quality and well-being for clients and their families.

THE COMMUNITY OUTREACH UNIT

On June 8, 2016, two Palestinian terrorists approached the Sarona Complex in Tel Aviv, the heart of Israeli culinary art, located about 150 yards from NATAL's center. Upon entering one of the complex's most popular restaurants, the terrorists opened submachine gunfire on restaurant clientele, killing three people and wounding 16. Some witnesses of the attack who remained physically unscathed suffered intense panic and anxiety. Within a few hours, NATAL's Helpline began receiving calls from civilians seeking emotional support, and from a large tour group of American students who were in the line of fire and present during the attack.

In the ensuing days, NATAL's Community Outreach Unit led sessions and workshops for emotional psychological first aid for the employees of the two restaurants that were attacked and the tour group participants who were in the vicinity. The sessions followed a protocol that includes psychoeducation to normalize the stress response, group reconstruction of the facts constituting the event, techniques for self-regulation of the physical arousal, and help in the recovery and continued functioning of individuals and organizations. Some people required continued support from the Helpline, and others were supported within NATAL's Clinical Unit. Several days after the attack, the Mobile Unit, which operates under the direction of the Community Outreach Unit, provided in-home interventions to survivors who, due to the severity of their distress, felt unable to leave their homes.

The Community Outreach Unit is the branch of NATAL whose role is to promote resilience in communities and individuals for stressful situations and emergencies to prevent or reduce pathogenic responses to traumatic events and promote healthy adaptation following trauma. The work of the unit takes place throughout the country and is unique in NATAL, as it is conducted in both the wake of disaster and its immediate and long-term aftermath. Building resilience is proactive universal work that focuses on building the community, strengthening existing coping mechanisms and resources, training professionals to provide emotional first aid, and drilling in positive psychology and readiness for emergencies.

The psychological distress triggered by exposure to a life threat and other atrocities related to political violence in Israel is manifold due to its continuing nature; therefore, the Community Outreach Unit employs an ecological viewpoint calling for attention to the various support systems that are accountable for an individual's well-being. Interventions of the unit combine proactive universal preventive interventions aimed at different levels of the ecosystems—family, communal, and social, alongside individually targeted clinical approaches. The unit identifies the strengths and resources available in the individual or community, joining with them and community leaders and professionals, as needed. It is always the goal of the Community Outreach Unit to try to approach from a position of humility, remembering that community leaders might have better insight into local needs.

Understanding that the clients' background, culture, society, and circumstances influence their reactions to the events is crucial. One of the most adverse mechanisms found for therapy during war was pathologizing those who exhibited normal reactions to adverse reality (Bosqui & Marshoud, 2018). In some circumstances, especially with continuous traumatic stress, individuals' needs are to adopt behaviors and defense mechanisms typified by high levels of alertness or restrictions (Eagle & Kaminer, 2013). Our therapists must have social and cultural awareness; learn to distinguish the normative from the pathogenic according to the circumstances; and accept a wide array of behaviors as normative, although hopefully temporary.

One example of our work is the "Safe Place" program for teachers and children in schools. During the course of multiple in-classroom workshops facilitated by a Community Outreach professional, teachers and students together learn about trauma, stress reactions, self-regulation, and relaxation techniques, as well as coping strategies via age-appropriate interactive presentations, group discussions, online exercises, and lesson plans. Years of the unit's experience with school programs revealed an improvement in the coping ability and self-efficacy among children, and a reduction of war- or terror-related distress (Berger, Gelkopf, & Heineberg, 2012; Gelkopf & Berger, 2009).

In times of emergency, and in its aftermath, we offer emotional first aid, preservation of strength, and restoration of balance to the communities. Our interventions are characteristically psychoeducational, where the main objective is normalization of response to stress and reduction of anxiety, along with guiding the population in adaptive behaviors and assisting in building positive, optimistic interpretations of responses to events. The individual and group interventions that were presented in the Sarona case description are typical examples of interventions conducted by group facilitators in the unit after emergency events.

In addition to single-incident attacks, there are regions of the country where the threat of rocket fire is omnipresent. This reality creates a situation where first responders, including emergency medical and mental health teams, are exposed to the same threats and losses as their clients. Since these organizations and professional groups face enormous pressure during emergencies, their risk of developing trauma symptoms, as well as secondary traumatization and professional burnout, is correspondingly high. Our "Helping the Helpers" program mitigates the burnout and distress resulting from working in a shared traumatic reality and reinforces their individual and organizational coping processes, a crucial factor in ensuring their continued functioning during periods of chaos and disorder.

PUBLIC RELATIONS DEPARTMENT

One of NATAL's main goals is to create visibility in public discourse for transparent traumatic wounds. NATAL addresses the social needs of trauma survivors and their families, thus creating legitimacy for seeking help. In doing so, the Public Relations Department actively promotes the positioning of NATAL as a leading professional knowledge source in the field, in Israel, and abroad. Undoubtedly, this complex challenge demands creativity and investment of resources.

Proactive media activities are designed to convey messages to wider target audiences through commercial communication channels. This includes television, radio, and newspaper ads; web banners; and advertising on social media networks. For example, each year, before Memorial Day, NATAL publishes a magazine titled *About Feelings*. The central theme is national trauma and ways of coping. One million copies of the issue are distributed as supplements to the major national newspapers.

Community Public Relation Activities

Community public relation activities include the following:

Running with Rami: Running groups for veterans with PTSD

Color-Run Race: A publicity and fund-raising event in which color is symbolic of creating visibility for the transparent wound (posttrauma) and the return to life.

Annual women's events: Focusing on a panel discussion emphasizing the gender aspects of the "world content" of NATAL

A children's play: Presenting *Kuntz and the Magic Mirror*, designed for early elementary schoolchildren, a community-educational tool created to mediate between young children and the struggle with unexpected situations. The play helps create resilience in existing educational settings, in familiar but exciting and artistic ways.

Safe Place: A designated website specifically designed for children in grades four through eight. It is a tool and platform to train teachers, educational consultants, and pupils in issues related to coping with stressful situations and emergencies, strengthening resources, and developing resilience.

MULTIDISCIPLINARY CENTER FOR TRAUMA-FOCUSED STUDIES AND TRAINING

Another important mission of NATAL is increasing trauma-related knowledge among the treating professions throughout the country. To this end, NATAL's Multidisciplinary Center for Trauma-Focused Studies and Training was established in 2007. The staff is comprised of leading Israeli professionals in the field of psychological trauma, who integrate knowledge and vast therapeutic experience, supervision, instruction, and research.

The NATAL model is reflected in the framework of the center's program: a multidisciplinary, humane, and holistic approach that is tailored to the specific needs of each client. Accordingly, it is important to integrate various therapeutic approaches and techniques, for instance, dynamic, narrative, cognitive, and behavioral therapies, along with others that address the somatic experiences of trauma and more.

The NATAL model enables a combination of interventions and continuity of care that finds expression in the study program and the various courses beginning with building resilience and preparedness. It accomplishes this end via intervention in communities exposed to traumatic events, providing a therapeutic response with the Helpline and clinical therapists using various approaches.

Owing to the importance of the subject, NATAL training has been recognized for continuing education credits to encourage civil servants to specialize in the field of trauma therapy. Since the establishment of the program a decade ago, thousands of students have been trained within its framework.

THE RESEARCH DEPARTMENT AS AN ORGANIZATIONAL RESOURCE

Data regarding efficacy and efficiency of services, as well as client characteristics and other needs, are necessary to generate growth in a large-scale organization like NATAL. The goals of NATAL's research and development (R&D) department are to monitor and continuously assess the effectiveness of interventions and services provided, as well as conduct large-scale studies to contribute to the scientific knowledge on trauma and resilience. The department has three objectives: 1) use the routinely collected data and empirical findings to improve services and better meet client needs; 2) provide data regarding the efficacy of NATAL's services to funding bodies and other stakeholders (e.g., policymakers); and 3) publish the results of the empirical studies, including services assessment (when relevant), in peer-reviewed journals, thus disseminating NATAL's professional work worldwide and advancing knowledge in the field of trauma and resilience.

Ongoing Assessments

NATAL's programs and interventions are routinely assessed by means of quantitative methods, namely, questionnaires based on standard assessment tools completed by clients and professionals. Data are collected on at least two time points (pre- and postintervention), whenever possible and relevant, and then undergo statistical analyses. Research reports presenting the results of these assessments are created routinely, in the form of data on specific populations or times, along with reports on individual clients.

An important aspect of the R&D work is sensitivity to clients' and professional staff's needs within the therapeutic/helping context of the organization. Thus, during data collection we take care not to impede the therapeutic process and make sure to minimize the burden on clients. Importantly, internal use of data for project evaluation is done in a constructive manner, with care being taken to prevent feelings of being "under scrutiny" by the professional staff. Research reports are triangulated with other formal and informal sources (e.g., client files).

The following are examples of routine assessments of specific programs and services: In the *clinical unit*, individual treatments are appraised using validated assessment scales (e.g., for posttraumatic stress or depression), as well as "soft" psychological measures (e.g., functional assessments and social support). Adult clients complete self-report questionnaires at the beginning of treatment, one year later, and/or at the end of treatment. Therapists also provide annual assessments. Children and parents complete questionnaires at the beginning and end of treatment.

An important element of the *Helpline* model is client anonymity and control (Gelkopf, Haimov, & Lapid, 2015). Trained volunteers, rather than clients, complete symptoms and functioning questionnaires at the onset of intervention, one year later, and/or at completion. Exposure and background data are also regularly collected and cross-tabulated with intervention-related data (e.g., length, type, and locus of intervention).

Community Outreach projects incorporate brief questionnaires administered to assess participant satisfaction in community projects. Long-term projects (e.g., resilience enhancement workshops) are assessed in depth, pre- and postintervention. Outcome measures are determined according to the program's aims and contents (e.g., professional self-efficacy).

Assessment of NATAL's Unique Intervention Models

NATAL's 20-year-long professional experience has led to the development of several unique intervention models aimed at reducing symptoms and building resiliency within various contexts and populations. Assessing the effectiveness of these models empirically is important for quality-enhancing purposes and possibly generalizing them to other populations. Such studies include, whenever applicable, control groups, randomization procedures, and advanced statistical analyses, and they are published in peer-reviewed journals. One example is a study evaluating the Helpline long-term intervention model, which was found to reduce symptomatology and improve functioning (Gelkopf, Haimov, & Lapid, 2015; Tamir & Haimov, 2005). A series of studies on the school-based interventions has found them to be effective in reducing symptomatology, improving functioning, and reducing intolerance in children and youth (Berger, Gelkopf, & Heineberg, 2012; Berger et al., 2016; Berger, Pat-Horencyk, & Gelkopf, 2007; Gelkopf & Berger, 2009). NATAL's program for reducing secondary traumatic stress and improving self-efficacy in nurses was also found to meet its goals effectively (Berger & Gelkopf, 2011).

Large-Scale Empirical Studies on National Trauma

Conducting empirical studies on the psychological implications of exposure to terror and war in Israeli society is necessary to pinpoint intervention needs and identify at-risk populations, as well as to advance the general scientific knowledge on trauma and its consequences. The R&D unit has conducted several such studies, mostly among civilians.

Large-scale nationally representative surveys have focused on mental health and resiliency reactions to terror and war in Israeli society (Bleich, Gelkopf, & Solomon, 2003; Bleich et al., 2006; Bleich, Solomon, & Gelkopf, 2013; Gelkopf, Solomon, & Bleich, 2013). Additional studies were conducted among such specific populations as soldiers (Bleich et al., 2008; Gelkopf, Berger, & Roe, 2016); older adults (Bleich et al., 2005; Palgi, Gelkopf, & Berger, 2015); women (Solomon, Gelkopf, & Bleich, 2005); the Arab minority (Gelkopf et al., 2008); people with disabilities (Berger et al., 2015; Shpigelman & Gelkopf, 2017); and urban versus rural populations (Gelkopf et al., 2012). Another large study conducted during the 2014 Israel–Gaza conflict used experience-sampling methodology to assess real-time reactions among an exposed sample with preconflict psychiatric diagnoses versus the general population (Gelkopf, Haimov, & Lapid, 2015; Gelkopf et al., in press; Greene, 2018; Greene et al., 2017; Greene et al., 2018; Lapid Pickman, Greene, & Gelkopf, 2017). We found that early reactions during war vary, are dynamic, and are affected by the context of the exposure. Symptoms, emotions, and cognitions develop differently throughout time, differ across various subgroups, and may be influenced by prior psychiatric diagnoses and gender.

CONCLUSION

The field of trauma treatment in Israel, as in throughout the world, is expanding, and the contribution of NATAL is unquestionable. As an organization committed to keeping this difficult subject on the agendas of the Israeli leadership and the general public, we are beginning to see significant progress in overall attitudes toward the legitimacy and understanding of post-trauma conditions.

NATAL organizes a broad spectrum of conferences, meetings, professional discussions, and academic research regarding trauma treatment and prevention. It also hosts international delegations from various countries interested in learning about the complex psychological impact of the ongoing conflict and its implications for life in Israel.

Twenty years have passed since the first announcement about opening a new center in Tel Aviv was made; the task has not yet been completed. Given that we are an organization that continues to develop and evolve, this is an opportunity for all of us to observe and assess our achievements thus far. At the same time as we are feeling great satisfaction and excitement, however, our reactions are mixed, as we understand that, in our present reality, we still have a long way to go.

QUESTIONS AND ANSWERS ABOUT NATAL

1. How does your work address what we have called the "whole person?" NATAL's therapeutic model is based on an extensive holistic view, applying various integrative therapeutic modalities that address

psychological, emotional, and somatic aspects, in a tailor-made fashion, and with emphasis on continuity of care. Interventions, which address the individual traumatic casualty, may include family members and the relevant community under threat.

2. What qualifications and training are needed to carry out your work? Professional staff (e.g., psychiatrists, psychologists, social workers, art therapists) are certified, licensed, and experienced. They have specific preparation and training for the various professional interventions, for instance, awareness of the social and cultural characteristics of the target populations. Helpline volunteers complete a seven-month training course that includes weekly four-hour sessions and three additional months of group supervision.
3. To what extent is your work evidence-based? Treatments and interventions are routinely evaluated for effectiveness using questionnaires pre- and postintervention. Some of NATAL's unique intervention models are empirically assessed, with controlled and randomized or quasi-randomized designs when applicable, and published in peer-reviewed journals.
4. How does your work reflect diversity, especially ethnic and gender diversity? NATAL staff work with all Israeli citizens, including Jews (religious and nonreligious) as well as Muslim and Christian Arabs, Druze, and Bedouins. This requires awareness and knowledge as to their specific social and cultural characteristics (e.g., gender issues), and the ability to adapt intervention modes accordingly.
5. What is the track record for those who have used your work? Our assessment studies repeatedly show a decrease in posttraumatic stress symptoms and other symptomatology, and an increase in functioning levels in clients who have undergone clinical treatments or Helpline interventions. Assessments of our community programs repeatedly show them to be effective in reducing emotional problems (in children) or burnout and secondary traumatic stress (in professionals), and increasing professional self-efficacy. Participants report confidence in their ability to use the skills and techniques learned.

ACKNOWLEDGMENTS

The following individuals contributed to this chapter (in alphabetical order): Dr. Itamar Barnea, Professor Avi Bleich, Gali Dagan, Yotam Dagan, Professor Marc Gelkopf, Dr. Sigal Haimov, Dr. Hana Himi, Liron Lapid Pickman, Dr. Tamar Lavie, Bina Levine, Ifat Morad, Rachel Oren, Professor Rivka Tuval-Mashiach, Gila Sella, and Sa'ar Uzieli.

REFERENCES

Berger, R., & Gelkopf, M. (2011). An intervention for reducing secondary traumatization and improving professional self-efficacy in well baby clinic nurses following war and terror: A random control group trial. *International Journal of Nursing Studies*, *48*, 601–10. doi: 10.1016/j.ijnurstu.2010.09.007.

Berger, R., Gelkopf, M., & Heineberg, Y. (2012). A teacher-delivered intervention for adolescents exposed to ongoing and intense traumatic war-related stress: A quasi-randomized controlled study. *Journal of Adolescent Health*, *51*, 453–61. doi: 10.1016/j.jadohealth.2012.02.011.

Berger, R., Gelkopf, M., Heineberg, Y., & Zimbardo, P. (2016). A school-based intervention for reducing posttraumatic symptomatology and intolerance during political violence. *Journal of Educational Psychology*, *108*(6), 761–71. doi: 10.1037/edu0000066.

Berger, R., Gelkopf, M., Versano-Mor, K., & Shpigelman, C. N. (2015). Impact of exposure to potentially traumatic events on individuals with intellectual disability. *American Journal of Intellectual and Developmental Disabilities*, *120*(2), 176–88. doi: 10.1352/1944-7558-120.2.176.

Berger, R., Pat-Horencyk, R., & Gelkopf, M. (2007). School-based intervention for prevention and treatment of elementary-pupils' terror-related distress in Israel: Quasi-randomized controlled trial. *Journal of Traumatic Stress*, *20*, 541–51. doi: 10.1002/jts.20225.

Bleich, A., Gelkopf, M., & Solomon, Z. (2003). Exposure to terrorism, stress-related mental health symptoms, and coping behaviors among a nationally representative sample in Israel. *Journal of American Medical Association*, *290*(5), 612–20. doi: 10.1001/jama.290.5.612.

Bleich, A., Gelkopf, M., Berger, R., & Solomon, Z. (2008). The psychological toll of the Intifada: Symptoms of distress and coping in Israeli soldiers. *Israel Medical Association Journal*, *10*(12), 873–79.

Bleich, A., Gelkopf, M., Melamed, Y., & Solomon, Z. (2005). Emotional impact of exposure to terrorism among young-old and old-old Israeli citizens. *American Journal of Geriatric Psychiatry*, *13*(8), 705–12. doi: 10.1176/appi.ajgp.13.8.705.

Bleich, A., Gelkopf, M., Melamed, Y., & Solomon, Z. (2006). Mental health and resiliency following 44 months of terrorism: A survey of an Israeli national representative sample. *BMC Medicine*, *4*(21), 1–11. doi: 10.1186/1741-7015-4-21.

Bleich, A., Solomon, Z., & Gelkopf, M. (2013). Editorial: Psychiatry and conflict. *Israel Journal of Psychiatry*, *100*, 78–80.

Bosqui, T. J., & Marshoud, B. (2018). Mechanisms of change for interventions aimed at improving the well-being, mental health, and resilience of children and adolescents affected by war and armed conflict: A systematic review of reviews. *Conflict and Health*, *12*(1), 15. doi: 10.1186/s13031-018-0153-1.

Clement, S., Schauman, O., Graham, T., Maggioni, F., Evans-Lacko, S., Bezborodovs, N., & Thornicroft, G. (2015). What is the impact of mental health-related stigma on help-seeking? A systematic review of quantitative and qualitative studies. *Psychological Medicine*, *45*(1), 11–27. doi: 10.1017/S0033291714000129.

Eagle, G., & Kaminer, D. (2013). Continuous traumatic stress: Expanding the lexicon of traumatic stress. *Peace and Conflict: Journal of Peace Psychology*, *19*(2), 85–99. doi: 10.1037/a0032485.

Gelkopf, M., & Berger, R. (2009). A school-based, teacher-mediated prevention program (ERASE-Stress) for reducing terror-related traumatic reactions in Israeli youth: A quasi-randomized controlled trial. *Journal of Child Psychology and Psychiatry*, *50*(8), 962–71. doi: 10.1111/j.1469-7610.2008.02021.x.

Gelkopf, M., Berger, R., Bleich, A., & Silver, R. C. (2012). Protective factors and predictors of vulnerability to chronic stress: A comparative study of four communities after seven years of continuous rocket fire. *Social Science & Medicine*, *74*(5), 757–66. doi: 10.1016/j.socscimed.2011.10.022.

Gelkopf, M., Berger, R., & Roe, D. (2016). Soldiers perpetrating or witnessing acts of humiliation: A community-based random sample study design. *Peace and Conflict: Journal of Peace Psychology*, *22*(1), 84–90. doi: 10.1037/pac0000154.

Gelkopf, M., Haimov, S., & Lapid, L. (2015). A community long-term hotline therapeutic intervention model for coping with the threat and trauma of war and terror. *Community Mental Health Journal*, *51*(2), 249–55. doi: 10.1007/s10597-014-9786-8.

Gelkopf, M., Lapid Pickman, L., Grinapol, S., Werbeloff, N., Carlson, E. B., & Greene, T. (2017). Peritraumatic reaction courses during war: Gender, serious mental illness, and exposure. *Psychiatry: Interpersonal and Biological Processes*, *80*(4), 382–98. doi: 10.1080/00332747.2017.1286893.

Gelkopf, M., Lapid Pickman, L., Carlson, E. B., & Greene, T. (In press). The dynamic relationship of peritraumatic phenomena: An experience sampling study during wartime. *Journal of Traumatic Stress.*

Gelkopf, M., Solomon, Z., Berger, R., & Bleich, A. (2008). The mental health impact of terrorism in Israel: A repeat cross-sectional study of Arabs and Jews. *Acta Psychiatica Scandinavica*, *117*(5), 369–80. doi: 10.1111/j.1600-0447.2008.01164.x.

Gelkopf, M., Solomon, Z., & Bleich, A. (2013). A longitudinal study of changes in psychological responses to continuous terrorism. *Israel Journal of Psychiatry and Related Sciences*, *50*(2), 100–109.

Greene, T. (2018). Do acute dissociation reactions predict subsequent posttraumatic stress and growth? A prospective experience sampling method study. *Journal of Anxiety Disorders*, *57*, 1–-6. doi: 10.1016/j.janxdis.2018.05.008.

Greene, T., Gelkopf, M., Grinapol, S., Werbeloff, N., Carlson, E., & Lapid, L. (2017). Trajectories of traumatic stress symptoms during conflict: A latent class analysis. *Journal of Affective Disorders*, *220*, 24–30. doi: 10.1016/j.jad.2017.05.036.

Greene, T., Gelkopf, M., Epskamp, S., & Fried, E. (2018). Dynamic networks of PTSD symptoms during conflict. *Psychological Medicine*, *48*(14), 2,409–17 doi: 10.1017/S0033291718000351.

Herman, J. L. (1994). *Trauma and recovery*. Tel Aviv, Israel: Am-Oved. [Hebrew]

Lapid Pickman, L., Greene, T., & Gelkopf, M. (2017). Sense of threat as a mediator of peritraumatic stress symptom development during wartime: An experience sampling study. *Journal of Traumatic Stress*, *30*(4), 372–80. doi: 10.1002/jts.22207.

Lester, D., & Rogers, J. R. (2012) *Crisis intervention and counseling by telephone and the internet* (3rd ed.). Springfield, IL: Charles C Thomas.

Lukens, E. P., & McFarlane, W. R. (2004). Psychoeducation as evidence-based practice: Considerations for practice, research, and policy. *Brief Treatment and Crisis Intervention*, *4*(3), 205–25.

Palgi, Y., Gelkopf, M., & Berger, R. (2015). The inoculating role of previous exposure to potentially traumatic life events on coping with prolonged exposure to rocket attacks: A lifespan perspective. *Psychiatry Research*, *227*(2/3), 296–301. doi: 10.1016/j.psychres.2015.03.020.

Rüsch, N., Hölzer, A., Hermann, C., Schramm, E., Jacob, G. A., Bohus, M., & Corrigan, P. W. (2006). Self-stigma in women with borderline personality disorder and women with social phobia. *Journal of Nervous and Mental Disease*, *194*(10), 766–73. doi: 10.1097/01.nmd.0000239898.48701.dc.

Shpigelman, C. N., & Gelkopf, M. (2017). The experiences and needs of individuals with disabilities exposed to chronic political violence. *Disability and Rehabilitation*, *39*(1), 23–35. doi: 10.3109/09638288.2016.1138557.

Solomon, Z., Gelkopf, M., & Bleich, A. (2005). Is terror gender-blind? Gender differences in reaction to terror events. *Social Psychiatry and Psychiatric Epidemiology*, *40*(12), 947–54. doi: 10.1007/s00127-005-0973-3.

Tamir, E., & Haimov, S. (2005). Telephone interventions after terrorist attacks. In E. Somer & A. Bleich (eds.), *Mental health in terror's shadow: The Israeli experience* (pp. 185–212). Tel Aviv, Israel: Ramot. [Hebrew]

Chapter Ten

Indigenous Healing Psychotherapy and Restorative Circles

Myron Eshowsky

Western psychotherapy's mainstream approaches to treating trauma focus primarily on individuals' problems and pathologies. These approaches often ignore the larger interpersonal and historical contexts that contribute to human thought and action, including the transmission—and healing—of trauma. Katz (2017) refers to the healing wisdom of indigenous people as the "first psychology." In his view, indigenous psychology focuses on issues of community building, interpersonal relations, and spiritual understanding. Most indigenous psychotherapies close the gap between individual and larger community contexts by viewing trauma in more holistic terms, seeing it as the loss of one's soul, along with the disconnection of relationships among self, others, and the larger circle of life. Indigenous people, in general, view the effects of trauma on an individual as being communal and spiritual, as well as personal; therefore, indigenous trauma treatments are seen as inseparable from spirituality: Healing restores intrapersonal, interpersonal, and communal connections, as well as those with all life forms.

This chapter focuses on the power of the circle, so to speak, inherent in most indigenous beliefs, through which we come to know ourselves and our wholeness. By extension, the wisdom of indigenous psychotherapies and the use of healing restorative circles and community ceremonies address the consequences of shared historical, multigenerational, and communal trauma. What follows is an exploration of the profound effects of how these concepts have resulted in communal healing when applied in culturally relevant ways to address trauma in the form of the impact of youth and gang violence.

HEALING RESTORATIVE JUSTICE CIRCLES

Since the 1970s, there has been considerable documentation in academic literature of the applications of restorative justice circles. Some writers have suggested that the starting point was the development of Victim Offender Mediation projects by the Mennonites in Canada (Alper & Nichols, 1981; Peachy, 2003; Umbreit, 1989). Others have indicated that restorative circles draw upon various cultural–spiritual and nonstate traditions, in which restorative justice is not so much an alternative to criminal prosecution as a way of living in faithfulness to what participants had already learned in life, identity, and spirit (Braithwaite, 1997; Marshall, 2001; Roach, 2000, 2002b; Van Ness & Strong, 1997; Weitekamp, 1993; Zher, 1990).

Sawatsky (2009) noted that the term *restorative justice circle* has no clear definition, creating a degree of confusion; however, the practice of restorative justice circles is clearly about restoring community connections. Sawatsky tentatively defined *healing justice* as a collective paradigm of imagination, usually drawing on ancient wisdom traditions seeking to find ways of surviving together—a process of structuring existence to reflect respect for life and a way of treating injuries as opportunities to transform suffering and the root causes of harm. At the same time, healing justice is a process of cultivating conditions of respectful living within the interrelated aspects of self, others, communities, social structures, environment, and "spirit" (Sawatsky, 2009, p. 39).

Johnstone and Van Ness (2007) delineated three overlapping conceptions of restorative justice as healing, each claiming to restore justice but with slightly different visions, goals, and sometimes methods. These three groupings are: encounter conception, reparative conception, and transformative conception. To come to some sort of definition, the authors identified six ingredients, proposing that at least one of them must be present for the process to be called *restorative justice*. These include the following:

1. Some sort of relatively informal process that aims to involve victims, offenders, and others connected to the harm in a discussion of what happened, what harm resulted, and what needs to be done to repair the harm.
2. An emphasis on empowering ordinary people whose lives had been affected by a wrongful act.
3. A process to promote the response of recognizing one's wrongdoing and taking responsibility to make amends for the harm caused.
4. A values-oriented system to promote desirable interactions between people, for example, respect for others, prevention of violence or coercion, and inclusion of all parties in the healing process.

5. An approach that gives significant attention to the harm done, the needs that resulted from that harm, and the tangible ways those needs can be addressed.
6. An emphasis on strengthening or repairing relationships between people and using those renewed relationships to resolve difficult situations. (p. 51)

Programs meeting several of those criteria might be the restorative justice circles used in South Africa and Cambodia, both of which drew upon their indigenous legacies to seek social restoration following decades of apartheid (in South Africa) or years of genocide (in Cambodia).

Braithwaite (2003) advocates the position that restorative justice can be an important strategy for advancing social justice, arguing that it may be able to lessen social injustices by reducing the impact of imprisonment. Indeed, incarceration often contributes to burdens of unemployment, debt, suicide, or rape, while restorative justice may give voice to decimated groups suffering from abuse.

The use of restorative justice circles in the United States can also be observed, especially with young people. Since the 1990s, school-based restorative justice has rapidly evolved (Gonzalez, 2016). A 2016 national survey found that schools in more than half the states in the United States, as well as the District of Columbia, were in some stage of implementing restorative justice (Gonzalez, 2016). This swift rise of restorative approaches in schools has transformed the field, allowing for a variety of approaches to be adapted, adopted, and interpreted in a diverse set of ways to fit the needs of each particular school community. While there is no consensual definition of *restorative approaches* in schools, there is academic consensus that it is grounded in indigenous traditions that emphasize interconnectedness and relationality to promote the well-being of all of its community members (Amstutz & Mullet, 2014; Lockhart & Zammit, 2005; Morrison, 2007; Zehr, 2005).

INDIGENOUS PSYCHOTHERAPY

Most indigenous psychotherapies are concerned with the welfare of all community members, with commitment to social justice as the aim and spirituality at its center. Indigenous psychotherapies, in general, emphasize understanding. Self-knowledge is pursued as a basis for knowing, so that being on a healing journey is seen as crucial for developing an accurate and fundamental self-knowledge. The focus is on communal knowing rather than individual prowess, since knowledge is meant to be shared. Indigenous psychotherapies attend to a whole way of living. Katz (2017) points out that Western models of psychology rarely discuss the fact that most non-Western cultures place topics of spirituality and healing at the center of their understandings of human nature. Indigenous peoples typically do not make clear distinctions between the *material* and the *spiritual*, thus giving spirituality a firm and recognizable place in the material flow of ordinary life. This perspective acknowledges that the *beyond* is also "within" us.

Indeed, spirituality is central to indigenous models of individual and community healing. Frank Clements (1932), who worked with indigenous peoples from throughout North America, understood indigenous healing in terms of *energetic transmissions* leading to 1) the removal of something that does not belong (e.g., spirit or object intrusion), and/or 2) the restoration of something that should be there and has gone missing (e.g., soul retrieval). These transmission categories include the following:

- Object intrusion: The belief that an object has intruded into the body. The object can invade the body as a result of some random event or can be placed there by someone wanting to cause suffering.
- Loss of soul: The belief that one's soul has been lost, misplaced, or stolen.
- Spirit intrusion: The belief that one's illness is caused by an outside entity invading the mind and body.
- Breech of taboo: Illness caused by the violation of a societal rule or custom.
- Sorcery: Illnesses that occur if someone with spiritual power willfully inflicts a physical, psychological, or spiritual malady on a person.

Through the knowledge, consideration, and diversity of community, it is believed that individuals achieve wholeness and self-identity, including a spiritual understanding of their selves, the communal systems, and the ways in which their unique natures and gifts are expressed and supported within the community as a whole. Clearly, indigenous psychotherapy is based on the belief that we are all connected and belong to a wider community. This principle of reciprocity is expressed by Judy Atkinson (Atkinson, Nelson, & Atkinson, 2010), a researcher of aboriginal descent (Jiman and Bjundjalung), who studies indigenous healing practices within Western trauma recovery processes:

> I will listen to you, share with you, as you listen to, share with me. Our shared experiences are different, but in the inner deep listening to, and quiet, still awareness of each other, we learn to grow together. In this we create community, and our shared knowledge and wisdom are expanded from our communication with each other. (pp. 17–18)

One indigenous approach to restorative justice is the use of community talking circles, which can be found in numerous societies throughout the world, for instance, those of the Dadirri (aboriginal peoples in Australia), the Dare' (the Shona tribe in South Africa and Zimbabwe), and the Sulha (in the Palestinian territories). Moreover, talking-stick restorative justice circles have been used for centuries in the First Nation tribes of Canada.

While it is widely accepted that restorative justice circles derive from indigenous practices, they are too often stripped of their spiritual richness. Anishinabe elder Danny Musqua shared that indigenous circles are "sacred ceremonies, more than just having people come together to talk, with an intent of healing" (in Katz, 2017, p. 413). In many indigenous traditions, the role of leading a ceremony is earned through the struggles of dedicated participation in previous ceremonies or a full apprenticeship. Katz (2017) observes that the circle, in the most ordinary sense, opens doors to strong and honest sharing, and is a therapeutic practice for everyone; however, Katz views Western adaptation of these circles as often removing the deeper indigenous context of healing the soul, while failing to convey spiritual understandings in their application.

Certain similarities in style and philosophy in the various cross-cultural models of the talking circle are recognizable. In general, all contain a belief that communities need to deal with their own harms rather than having them diverted to foreign systems. Healing is seen as starting with the individual within the context of a supportive community. It is, in short, seen as communal; when one person is hurt, everyone is affected, so the healing cannot be limited to the afflicted person. Another shared core belief is a shift from symptoms to root causes—that is, in many cases, responding meaningfully to presenting symptoms means the group has to dig deeper to find the root causes. These may be childhood sexual abuse or traumas resulting from colonialism, civil wars, and domestic violence. Most societies believe that they must heal the generations of trauma and bring it to an end to bring about health for the generations ahead.

In general, restorative justice circles have certain structural styles in common, namely the following:

- An opening ritual that affirms everyone's interconnection and calls on the help of a higher power, the ancestors, and the wisdom of the Elders
- A general theme of the day proposed by a group leader, elder, or the group itself
- *Deep listening* with all of the senses, during which each person has an opportunity to share without disruption, criticism, or judgment
- The holding of a stick, feather, or stone when it is time to talk
- Speaking from the heart and connecting words to topics others have discussed that struck a chord within the current speaker

- Some sort of ritualized closing that again affirms everyone's interconnection

EVIDENCE-BASED RESEARCH AND ITS LIMITATIONS

Gonzalez, Sattler, and Buth (2018) note three strands of applied research approaches in the assessment of restorative justice:

1. *Quantitative research* aimed at being responsive to discipline and reduced reliance on punitive practices.
2. *Qualitative assessment* of associated outcomes and benefits of restorative approaches in such areas as improved school safety, increased school connectedness, conflict resolution skills development, and social emotional learning.
3. *Research* analyzing the process and development of such approaches as whole-school methods seeking to improve relationships among students, teachers, and staff; strengthening equity; and using culturally sensitive practices. (pp. 2–4)

Morrison, Blood, and Thorsborne (2005) describe such whole-school restorative practices as creating a system with primary, secondary, and tertiary tiers that foster high levels of support for collaboration:

Tier 1: Doing things *with* someone as opposed to doing things *to* or *for* someone. Primary-tier interventions engage every member and focus on developing skills for shared emotional support and competencies, thereby creating a restorative culture grounded in shared values and skills.

Tier 2: Applying to specific individuals in the community by repairing harms.

Tier 3: Drawing in those who have chronic behavioral problems and need the most intensive intervention, involving a wider cross-section of the school community.

A number of indigenous researchers have been quite critical of Western-style evidence-based research. Judy Atkinson (Atkinson, Nelson, and Atkinson, 2010) makes the point that Western researchers often overlook the knowledge that indigenous people have of their own challenges and needs. She and Native American psychologist Eduardo Duran (2006) describe the resistance of an indigenous community to an imposition from the outside of what was to be researched and how the research was to be framed. Duran (2006) shares his early experience working with native people, using research questionnaires that made sense from his Western academic perspective yet obtained no useful responses from the community he was trying to assess. He came to believe that researchers need to know the community they are studying and work collaboratively with it to gain meaningful cooperation. Freire (1996), educator and author of the classic book *Pedagogy of the Oppressed*, argues that the knowledge and wisdom of oppressed groups provide the most credible information regarding solutions to the problems they face. Freire made the case that those being researched should be cocreators of the knowledge to be acquired.

Duran and Firehammer (2017), Judy Atkinson (Atkinson, Nelson, & Atkinson, 2010), Sawatsky (2009), and Smith (2012) point out the need for culturally responsive models for dealing with both trauma and research. Duran and Firehammer (2017) argue that, unless research is deeply rooted in the lifeworld metaphor of the culture, effectiveness is limited, at best, and more trauma will occur, at worst. Smith (2012) argues that the indigenous view has a "different epidemiological tradition, which frames the way people see their world, the way they organize themselves in it, the questions they ask, and the solutions they seek" (p. 190). In describing the research approaches she used to study healing restorative circles in the treatment of trauma among indigenous people of Australia, Judy Atkinson (Atkinson, Nelson, & Atkinson, 2010) refers to it as a *narrative approach* that could be incorporated into Western research methodologies. The elements of this approach are as follows:

- Consciousness-raising: The value given to community processes to raise awareness within the researcher and the researched (both seen as inclusive).
- Participatory action: The contribution that people make in their activities of relating, defining, and narrating together their own life experiences. All parts are recognized as essential to the whole.
- Phenomenology: The understanding of the relationship between the inner world of an individual and the outer world of social relationships. (p. 16)

Bryant-Davis and Ocampo (2005) point out that most diagnostic systems for posttraumatic stress disorders fail to account for chronic interpersonal trauma and discrimination, and their effect on minority populations. Shelton and Delgado-Romero (2011) note that many who are subjugated within the dominant American culture often experience microaggressions and other forms of societal trauma throughout their lifespan. Although there is a considerable evidence base for standard PTSD treatments—e.g., Bradley et al. (2005)—conflicting data indicate that exposure, cognitive-behavioral, and EMDR therapies actually have highly variable nonresponse and dropout rates (Cloitre et al., 2002; Schottenbauer et al., 2008). Moreover, it is worth noting that much of the evidence focuses on symptom reduction of DSM-defined outcomes of PTSD without accounting for the differential effects on types of trauma (Bisson et al., 2007).

Two major studies of restorative circles that address the communal trauma of indigenous people (Atkinson, 2015, in Australia, and Ross, 2006, in Canada) found similar results. Traumatic violence fragments people's sense of themselves, their identity, their family, and their community. Violence shatters the loving and enduring connections of family and community that provide structure to people's lives. Studies using participant self-reports, along with public health data showing reductions in community violence, suicide, and reported alcohol/other substance abuse, showed the following:

- Circles built positive feelings of self-worth, an increased sense of belonging, and a shared sense of community.
- Circles helped participants make sense of their own trauma stories in relationship to the collective communal story.
- The old story of traumatic violence was deconstructed, and a new story of healing and life-meaning was built.

Both of these studies cited and confirmed Brave Heart-Jordan's finding (1995) that education about historical trauma leads to increased awareness about trauma, its impacts, and related grief effects. Duran et al. (1998) found that reducing the grief effects in the world of indigenous people led to positive identity and a commitment to continued healing. These findings are significant, given the high rates of dropout from conventional Western psychological treatment. Indeed, Duran et al. (1998) suggest that treatments tailored to cultural and community responses to trauma are vital to break the distrust of most Western psychotherapy treatments.

Case Example

For several years in the 1990s and early 2000s, I led restorative healing circles in the Allied Drive neighborhood of Madison, Wisconsin. There were growing concerns related to youth and gang violence, and neighborhood frustration with the lack of any services addressing youth. At that time, the neighborhood was made up of two distinct gang groups divided along racial lines: Southeast Asian (primarily Khmer and Hmong) and African American. Family and communal traumas characterized members of both groups. The Southeast Asian families brought with them trauma from the Vietnam War and the Khmer Rouge regime. The parents, by and large, did not speak English, while the children spoke English but not the language of their adult parents. Boys, 5 years of age and older, were largely left to their own devices, as had been the practice in villages back home. This put the boys at risk to be influenced by street life, and they were often bereft of adult authority. Most of the African American families had moved from Chicago to get away from the violence there, only to see it recreated in their new neighborhoods.

When they were invited to engage in restorative healing circles, most neighborhood and community service providers commonly accepted the idea that boys older than 12 were already unreachable. The attitudes of the adults were increasingly moving toward control and punishment as the way to change the situation in the neighborhood. I gave a presentation to parents and community service organizations about the difference between indigenous healing treatments and the dominant themes of Western culture, offering them the indigenous perception that everything is connected and that community life is a priority. From this perspective, young people were seen as an expression of their community. Eshowsky (1999) contrasts this with the more individualistic notions of Western culture in which the individual operates separately from the community. The presentation focused on reclaiming family and community roots, and looking at these community issues as also being spiritual ones.

I convinced the adult community to try a different approach. Healing restorative circle facilitators began to walk the neighborhood on a regular basis to encounter youth on the streets. My student assistants and I would talk about healing. We used their own language for trauma, like "There's been a lot of s**t going down." We spoke of "squashing it," which was their way of talking about interrupting conflict before it turned to violence. Our position was that it was more important to step into the worldview in which these young people operated than to offer "expert opinions" that diminished their own understandings.

Many of the youth asked about ghosts, since they had stories about friends who had been killed and ghosts were part of their cultural tradition. Most wanted to talk about traumatizing events they had witnessed and, in some cases, the upsetting dreams they had afterward. After a few weeks of informal circles on the streets, we began our first formal talking circles with a mix of youth from both gangs to process the violence, loss, and trauma they had experienced.

A key factor in the circles becoming places of nondisruptive deep listening was identifying the natural leaders/healers of the gangs and winning them over to engagement. Although the needs and issues of the two gangs were different in significant ways, related to differences in their native countries' historical trauma, by and large the two gangs were not in competition with one another.

The key person in the Southeast Asian youth gang was Chou. He was clearly the largest of the boys, with a reputation for being a fighter. In a conversation with him, he shared with me his love of fighting. As I asked more and more questions, it was clear he was releasing his own pain by giving it to others. During one of our circles, we took a group break; while Chou was outside, someone came in to have a fight with him. Chou bloodied the rival gang member's nose, as some of the boys came to tell me once the conflict had ended. After the fight, Chou was clearly morose and withdrawn. When I asked him how he was feeling, he simply said, "Can we do that soul healing stuff you talk about?" We did a healing ceremony for all the boys (not just Chou), with the goal of helping them feel more centered in their bodies. Afterward, Chou was clearly feeling much better. From that point onward, he made sure other gang members came to the talking circles.

The importance of *deep listening* is crucial in these groups. So many of the youth in the circle did not feel heard. Yet, they knew what their problems were and what they needed. The absence of being listened to by adults clearly exacerbated issues about being "respected." Often the boys would claim that their issues were so formidable that only "God" could fix them. Sometimes we would engage in group spiritual visualization related to a theme they would identify. In one case, it was "how to find peace." Strikingly, many of the African American youth came back with images of the wounds of slavery. "We don't want to be slaves no more," was a common refrain. One of them imagined dancing out the conflicts of the slaves. The strongest thread connecting their visualizations was the theme that we were to create a ritual to heal the wounds of slavery—that is, directly address the influence of historical trauma.

It was suggested that we create a ritual of dancing to bring healing for the slaves. Some of us drummed for those who volunteered to dance. As the dancing began, it was aggressive and fast. Then some of the dancers started to shake, as if being taken over by a spiritual force. A rhythmic chant began to emerge, and the dancers shifted into a different mode. Still strong and fierce, it lacked its earlier aggressiveness, which showed that the energy was shifting or transforming. Often, what might happen in this sort of context of dancing as healing is that those in the circle would dance the spirit of our focus. In this case, it was the trauma of slaves, many of whom were ancestors as well. Thus, the dance spiritually shifted from an energy of trauma into an energy of healing. More of the boys were encouraged to join the dance, which also increased the power of the ceremony, until it came to a natural resolution or close. The intent was to build a positive container of belonging as a community.

Later, during the talking circle, the dancers described feeling as if something had taken them over. They wanted the group leaders to tell them what had happened. We discussed the notion of helping spirits and ancestors to bring healing. This stirred a dialogue of how most carried a negative view of family and how much they thought the ancestors would be like their families. I talked about how the ancestors had been here, how they knew the struggles we have here on Earth, and how they wanted to be of help. These ceremonies had the positive effect of encouraging circle members to bring more gang members to the talking circles.

Throughout time, we received feedback from the high school indicating increased school attendance and decreased criminal justice issues involving talking-circle attendees. Community incidents of violence were reduced by 17% in our first year per local police incident reports, and, with the aid of the youths, we were able to sponsor a number of community events. The gangs adopted the ideal of random acts of kindness in the neighborhood, of being of service to the greater community. We organized a community-wide picnic, along with a community Peace Tree ceremony. Because of the large number of Southeast Asian refugees in the community, we were able to have Hmong and Khmer shamans participate, talk with the boys, and lead a protection ceremony. Circle members would say to us, "My uncle does things like you are doing," and they would take us to meet their elders. These meetings won their endorsement and involvement in what we were doing. I had personally been initiated in the Shona traditions of healing (Zimbabwe), and my mentor agreed to come and work with me. We walked through the neighborhood and talked with the people on the streets. Bringing healers of their own heritage and creating their own rituals that mimicked rituals from their ancestral homeland had a positive effect on the boys in terms of addressing the historical legacy that had been lost.

Ironically, two related but separate events undercut the progress that was made. During this time, the police arrested a key African American gang member, known by his street name as Big Paul, for dealing drugs. Big Paul, who was respected by all the gangs, played a key role in interrupting events when they seemed about to turn violent. The young people called him when conflicts were emerging, and he would moderate the conflicts and cool them down. Despite appeals to the authorities not to send Big Paul away, he was sentenced to the state prison. Neighborhood violence began to rise in the absence of Big Paul's influence. This became a background for the city's decision to tear down some of the buildings in which people were living, dispersing families to new neighborhoods. Hence, we lost the feeling of community cohesion and trust we had built as people were dispersed throughout the city. We were not able to continue the program due to the fragmentation that followed.

CONCLUSION

Unlike more conventional Western therapeutic approaches to trauma, indigenous psychotherapy and restorative justice circles understand and heal trauma on individual, communal, and spiritual levels. A strongly held indigenous belief is that people heal in community. Healing is not so much the treatment of diseases and disabilities as it is an educational process of self-discovery and reconnection. Restorative circles provide a culturally safe environment for people to do the deeper work needed to change their lives.

This process of exploration is both individual and collective, with an emphasis on expressing the deeper feelings that have been suppressed and unrecognized. In doing so, individually and collectively, the circle is able to make sense of the trauma stories that have previously seemed senseless. Restorative circle work, particularly that addressing shared communal and historical trauma, reveals an understanding of layers of loss and grief. Healing is seen as a process of moving through the pain and transforming the pain into a new story and a sense of freedom.

Training in the facilitation of restorative circles has expanded, particularly in their use in schools and the criminal justice system (Gonzalez et al., 2018). As a result, a growing collection of evidence supports the effectiveness of restorative circles to reduce truancy, school violence, and bullying in the schools, as well as recidivism in the criminal justice system. Research results support findings of increased school performance and community participation (Gonzalez et al., 2018). Online searches reveal that a large number of U.S. colleges and universities now offer training in restorative justice circles, particularly in the fields of social work, education, and law.

Unfortunately, I discovered anecdotally that a number of graduate schools that had initiated group work no longer teach it. A contributing factor cited was that insurance funding favored individual treatment. In such cases as addiction treatment, even where funding exists for group work, it is at a much lower reimbursement rate, which discourages the initiation of these services. Private training, particularly of volunteers for such community-based restorative justice circles as victim/offender conferencing and drug courts, is, however, available in all 50 states and the District of Columbia (Gonzalez et al., 2018).

Nonetheless, sensitivity to cultural misappropriation and use remains of concern. Dobkin de Rios (1994) and Prayag Grish et al. (2015) have been critical of rapid spiritual seeking in ayahuasca tourism. An understanding of indigenous wisdom that informs restorative circles is developed through respectful relationships and participation in ceremonies throughout time, not by time-limited exposure similar to a professional training workshop. Eduardo Duran has cautioned about the importance of applying a critical eye to the process of colonialization and its impact on native peoples. Methods like restorative circle work are seen not as specific techniques, but rather as a part of a holistic way of being with the world. "Healers who are part of the original communities do not pretend they are beyond the frailties of being human. The community acknowledges their wounding and healing process, which can provide a bridge of compassion needed in the healing of patients" (Duran, 2006, p. 6).

REFERENCES

Alper, B. S., & Nichols, L. T. (1981). *Beyond the courtroom: Programs in community justice and conflict resolution*. Lexington, MA: Lexington Books.

Amstutz, L. S., & Mullet, J. H. (2014). *The little book of restorative discipline for schools: Teaching responsibility, creating caring climates*. New York: Good Books.

Atkinson, J. (2015). *Trauma Trails recreating song lines: The transgenerational effects of trauma in indigenous Australia*. North Melbourne, Australia: Spinifex Press.

Atkinson, J., Nelson, J., & Atkinson, C. (2010). Trauma, transgenerational trauma, and effects of community well-being. In N. Purdie, P. Dudgeon, & T. Walker (eds.), *Working together: Aboriginal and Torres Strait Islander mental health and well-being* (pp. 135–44). Canberra, Australia: Australian Health and Welfare.

Bing, L. (1994). *Do or die*. New York: HarperCollins.

Bisson, J. I., Ehlers, A., Matthews, R., Pilling, S., Richards, D., & Turner, S. (2007). Psychological treatments for chronic posttraumatic stress disorder: Systematic review and meta-analysis. *British Journal of Psychiatry*, *190*(2), 97–104.

Bradley, R., Greene, J., Russ, E., Dutra, L., & Westen, D. (2005). A multidimensional meta-analysis of psychotherapy for PTSD. *American Journal of Psychiatry*, *162*, 214–27.

Braithwaite, J. (1997). Assessing immodest theory and a pessimistic theory. In M. Torrey (Ed), *Crime and justice: Annual review of research* (vol. 25, pp. 54–66). Chicago, IL: University of Chicago Press.

Braithwaite, J. (2003) Restorative justice and social justice. In E. McLaughlin, R. Ferguson, C. Hughes, & L. Westmorland (eds.), *Restorative justice: Cultural issues* (pp. 54–66). London, UK: Sage.

Brave Heart-Jordan, M. Y. H. (1995). *The return to the Sacred Path: Healing historical trauma and historical unresolved grief amongst the Lakota*. Doctoral dissertation. Northampton, MA: Smith College of Social Work.

Bryant-Davis, T., & Ocampo, C. (2005). Racist incident-based trauma. *Counseling Psychologists*, *33*(4), 479–500.

Clements, F. (1932). Primitive concepts of disease. *Archeology and Ethnography*, *32*(2), 85–252.

Cloitre, M., Koenen, K. C., Cohen, L. R., & Han, H. (2002). Skills training in affective and interpersonal regulation following exposure: A phase-based treatment for PTSD. *Journal of Consulting and Clinical Psychology*, *70*(5), 1,067–74.

Dobkin de Rios, M. (1994). Drug tourism in the Amazon. *Anthropology of Consciousness*, *5*(1), 90–109.

Duran, E. (2006). *Healing the soul wound: Counseling with American Indians and other native peoples*. New York: Teachers College Press.

Duran, E., & Firehammer, J. (2017). Injury where blood does not flow. In S. Stewart, R. Moodley, & A. Hyatt (eds.), *Indigenous cultures and mental health counseling: Four directions for integration with counseling psychology* (pp. 107–24). New York: Routledge.

Duran, E., Duran, B., Brave Heart-Jordan, M. Y. H., & Yellow Horse-Davis, S. (1998). Healing the American Indian soul wound. In Y. Danieli (ed.), *International handbook of multigenerational legacies of trauma* (pp. 341–54). New York: Plenum.

Eshowsky, M. (1999). Community shamanism: Youth, violence, and healing. *New Village: Building Sustainable Cultures Journal*, *1*(1), 28–33.

Eshowsky, M. (2016). History that never ends: Healing transgenerational trauma in community life. In T. Gaillard (ed.), *Shamanism, ancestors, and transgenerational integration: Traditional wisdom and contemporary practices* (pp. 77–98). Geneva, Switzerland: Ecoditions Press.

Freire, P. (1972/1996). *Pedagogy of the oppressed*. London: Penguin.

Gonzalez, T. (2016). Restorative justice from the margins to the center: The emergence of the new norm in school discipline. *Howard University Law Journal*, *60*(1), 267–308.

Gonzalez, T., Sattler, H., & Buth, A. J. (2018). New directions in whole-school restorative justice implementation. *Conflict Resolution Quarterly*, *38*, 1–14.

Grish, P., Mura, M., Hall, M., & Fontaine, J. (2015). Drug or spirituality seekers? Consuming ayahuasca. *Annals of Tourism Research*, *52*, 1–3.

Jabbour, E. J. (1996). *Sulha: Palestinian traditional peacemaking process*. Jerusalem: House of Hope Publications.

Johnstone, G., & Van Ness, D. W. (2007). Restorative justice: An overview. In G. Johnstone & D. W. Van Ness (eds.), Handbook of restorative justice (pp. 5–24). Cullampton, UK: Willan.

Katz, R. (2017). *Indigenous healing psychology: Honoring the wisdom of the First Peoples*. Rochester, VT: Healing Arts Press.

Lockhart, A., & Zammit, L. (2005). *Restorative justice: Transforming society*. Toronto: Inclusion Press.

Marshall, C. D. (2001). *Beyond retribution: A New Testament vision for justice, crime, and punishment*. Grand Rapids, MI: William B. Eerdmans.

Morrison, B. (2007) *Restoring safe school communities: A whole-school response to bullying*. Sydney, Australia: Federation Press.

Morrison, B., Blood, P., & Thorsborne, M. (2005). Practicing restorative justice in school communities: The challenge of culture change. *Public Organization Review*, *5*(4), 335–57.

Peachey, D. (2013). The Kitcher Experiment. In G. Johnstone (ed.), *Restorative justice reader* (pp. 178–90). Cullampton, UK: Willan.

Prayag, G., Mura, P., Hall, C. M., & Fontaine, J. (2015). Spirituality, drugs, and tourism. *Tourism Recreation Research, 41*, 1–12.

Roach, K. (2000). Changing punishment at the turn of the century, restorative justice on the rise, *Canadian Journal of Criminology, 42* (3), 249–79.

Ross, R. (2006). *Returning to the teachings: Exploring aboriginal justice*. Toronto: Penguin.

Sawatsky, J. (2009). *The ethic of traditional communities and the spirit of healing justice: Studies from Hollow Water, the Iona Community, and Plum Village*. Philadelphia, PA: Jessica Kingsley.

Schottenbauer, G., & Arnkoff, G. (2008). Non response and dropout rates in action studies on PTSD: review and methodological considerations, *Psychiatry, 71* (2), 134–68.

Shelton, K., & Delgado-Romero, E. A., (2011), Sexual orientation micro-aggressions, *Journal of Counseling Psychology, 58* (2), 210–21.

Smith, L. T. (2012). *Decolonizing methodologies: Research and indigenous peoples*. New York: St. Martin's.

Umbreit, M. S. (1989). Crime victims seeking fairness, not revenge: Toward restorative justice. *Federal Probation Journal, 53*(3), 52–57.

Van Ness, D., & Strong, K. H. (1997). *Restoring justice*. Cincinnati, OH: Anderson Publishing.

Van Ness, D. W., & Strong, K. (1997). *Restorative justice practice*. Washington, D.C.: Justice Fellowship.

Weitekamp, E. (1993). Reparative justice, *European Journal on Criminal Policy and Research, 1* (1), 70–93.

Zehr, H. (2005). *Changing lenses: A new focus for crime and justice*. Scottsdale, PA: Herald Press.

Zehr, H. (1990). *Mediating victim offender conflict: The victim offender reconciliation program*. Akron, PA: Mennonite Central Committee.

Chapter Eleven

Whole-Person Approaches in Individual and Communal Healing of Trauma

Steve S. Olweean

While disastrous psychoemotional trauma can be triggered by a variety of events, both natural and human-caused, the most devastating and lasting are those intentionally perpetrated at the hands of others. When such a disaster is inflicted on an entire society, it can permeate every level of the community to place its members at even more risk of prolonged and debilitating suffering (Butler, Panzer, & Goldfrank, 2003).

Particularly in societies with massive and growing at-risk populations and underdeveloped or seriously compromised mental health service systems, the challenges are monumental. Further complicating the situation are issues we see as not uncommon when dealing with catastrophic events impacting entire communities, especially in developing societies.

Humanitarian aid to communities suffering from such catastrophes historically tends to focus more on the most visible and concrete needs, for example, food, clothing, shelter, medical assistance, and so on, most often to the neglect of less immediately visible psychoemotional wounds (Olweean, 2003). Over time, such wounds can become embedded in the personal and collective consciousness and identity, to be passed on to future generations as inherited trauma (Milroy & Zubrick, 2005).

At the same time, emergency treatment providers who do attempt to address mental health needs—particularly those coming from outside the community and culture—may tend to approach these recovery needs from an overly specialized, standardized, and culturally biased perspective that seeks to frame the individual and communal experience within the specific models with which they are most familiar and effective in using (Wessels & Montei-

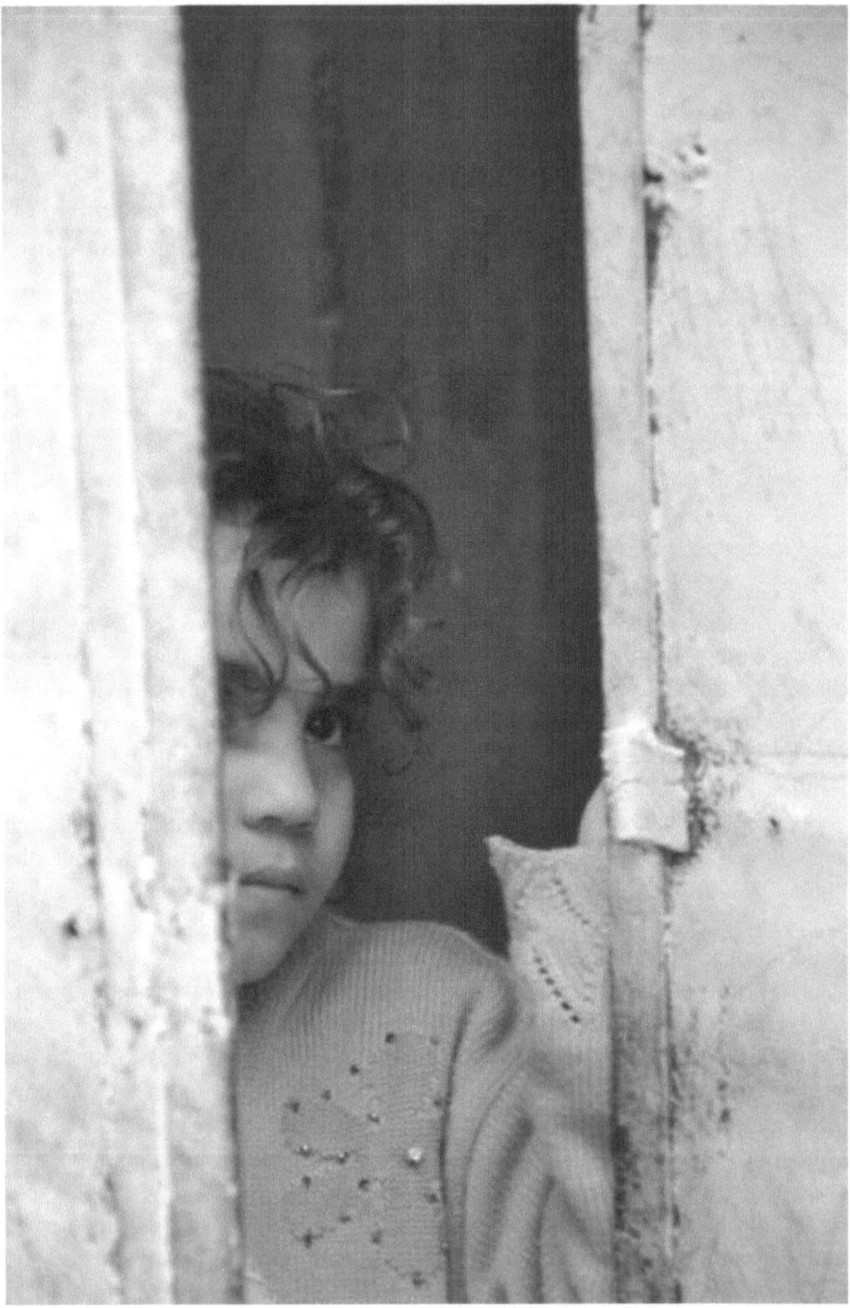

Figure 11.1. CBI outreach services to Syrian refugee children. Amman, Jordan.

ro, 2001). They can also tend to focus more exclusively on purely psycho-emotional treatment needs to the exclusion of those that are more concrete but essential to day-to-day stability and survival (Wessels & Monteiro, 2003).

When local treatment skill resources are significantly lacking, the number of outside therapists available at any one time compared to the immense size of the local victim population is also limited; moreover, treatment is only temporarily available, because the foreign therapists eventually leave the community, taking their services with them. Thus, there is only a minimal impact, at best, on the current level of need in conditions where the need is growing and becoming more chronic (Silove, Ventevogel, & Rees, 2017).

Current models and methods in the field of contemporary mental health designed for individual, family, and small group treatment are clearly inadequate for addressing trauma at a large societal scale. Even in the face of obvious implications for the future of an entire community imbedded with unhealed trauma, this lack of readily available means to treat systemic trauma at the communal level may lead to reduced expectations for communal healing, or even for addressing the need, along with an attitude that it is "too big to heal" (Davis, Pinderhughes, & Williams, 2015).

We have found that the effects of profound trauma due to war and violence on individuals and their communities create exceptional challenges to mental health treatment. These are simply not adequately addressed by highly specialized, standardized, and culturally limited approaches, an overly narrow focus on types of recovery needs, and attempts by small numbers of outside therapists to treat temporarily massive numbers of victims on an individual, family, and small group basis.

Our assessment, therefore, is that a culturally sensitive, whole-person approach is the most useful in promoting a broader, more in-depth understanding and response to the healing and recovery process, as well as a greater benefit to both an individual's and an entire community's overall quality of life, stability, and sense of meaning, purpose, dignity, and identity.

FOCUS OF THIS CHAPTER

The focus of this chapter is to share observations and programs that have grown out of working directly with communities in developing societies that have been experiencing pervasive and catastrophic communal trauma by doing the following:

- Identifying key interrelated factors that influence healing and recovery outcomes

- Illustrating the Catastrophic Trauma Recovery (CTR) Model, as an integrated, holistic, and local capacity-building model informed by these factors for promoting individual and communal healing, renewal, and post-trauma growth
- Offering the example of the Social Health Care (SHC) training and treatment program based on this model currently being used to address the Syrian refugee crisis in the Middle East

KEY FACTORS

During more than two decades of the Common Bond Institute (CBI) working with societies in regions of conflict that have produced countless refugees, we have identified four key factors that substantially influence the potential for adequately healing and recovering from community-wide trauma and loss. These factors are as follows:

1. Whether the multifaceted and interacting nature of the full experience is acknowledged and attended to.
2. Whether both the quantitative and qualitative dimensions of the individual and communal experience of loss and wounding are attended to.
3. Whether the experience is addressed within the cultural context and at both the individual and communal levels.
4. Whether the community is equipped with the capacity to be the primary provider of its own healing and recovery.

Multiple Interacting Aspects of the Experience

Victimized populations can face numerous significant stressors, often concentrated within the same period of time. These stressors can relate to both basic daily living and existential needs, overlap, interact, and merge to magnify the overall power and durability of the loss experience.

The most immediate example of working with Syrian refugees, in particular, since 2011 has led us to consider a number of compounding stress factors. These include the following:

- psycho-emotional and physical trauma
- general health decline
- loss of loved ones and close social relationships
- loss of community cohesion and sense of belonging
- loss of individual and communal esteem, confidence, and dignity
- loss of civil society and institutional support systems
- loss of individual, family, and sociocultural role and identity

- loss of home and worldly possessions
- loss of education, occupation, socioeconomic means, and self-sufficiency
- persecution, exploitation, and diminished civil rights as a marginalized refugee
- for those settling in lands far from their home culture, culture shock in an often new, foreign, and uninviting society

The emotional and psychological toll of multiple disrupting life changes can cause substantial strains and drains on the energy, stamina, and internal resources required of a person to adjust adequately to these changes. When they occur within a brief period, or essentially all at once, and particularly when acute trauma is present, the cumulative effect can be incapacitating. Being able to regain some degree of balance and stability in a person's original sense of security, familiarity, and belonging better allows for a steadier, more successful recovery and adjustment to difficult conditions and disruptive life changes. Given this, support of full recovery requires acknowledging and, where feasible, offering the assistance required to respond to as many of these elements as possible.

Quality of the Experience

A second key influencing factor has to do with what "type" of needs are attended to, including both the quantitative and qualitative elements of loss and wounding. While the quantity of stressors plays a significant role in creating difficult and compounding obstacles for those struggling to recover to a previous level of daily functioning, the qualitative impact of severe psychoemotional harm on the individual and, in turn, the community they make up, is most often the deepest, longest lasting, and most difficult wound to recover from. The presence of such harm can also amplify the overall stress of major losses and life changes.

Profound trauma can permeate every dimension of an individual's reality; and along the way, previously secure positive beliefs can be fundamentally shaken, or even shattered, to be replaced by debilitating and damaging negative beliefs and fragmented perceptions of reality that color every aspect of day-to-day life from that point onward. If their trauma is unhealed, the underlying meaning an individual attaches to the experience can galvanize into a system of beliefs about themselves, others, the world, and their place in it that perpetuates the wounding and a victim narrative into their future, and potentially that of their children (Olweean, 2002).

On a communal level, the process is even more complex. Trauma at a large scale, penetrating every level of a society and going unhealed, can become embedded in the group ethos to create shared and socially reinforced legacies of unresolved communal trauma and victim identities that extend into future generations as transgenerational trauma (Volkan, 1998). The dynamics of a reciprocal relationship between communal trauma and the individual traumas of its members further complicates matters, as is discussed later in this chapter.

"Psychological and emotional injuries may in fact be the most enduring effects of war and violence, yet historically they are the least addressed in terms of either individual or communal recovery" (Olweean, 2003, p. 271). Treating large civilian populations suffering from pervasive trauma poses unique challenges for contemporary treatment models. In societies where human services are seriously underdeveloped or absent, or where the integrity of the existing social support system has been critically weakened, these challenges can be all the more overwhelming (Olweean, 2003). Indeed, we find that, when there are a significant number of traumatized members of a community, approaches that do not also include addressing the community as a whole are likely to be limited and less than adequate, falling short of their goals.

Cultural Context of the Experience

A third influencing factor is the cultural and spiritual context of the trauma and loss experience. It is important to frame both the experience and the various approaches to treatment and recovery directly within this context.

Applying perspectives, models, and methods from outside that are not adapted to or reflective of the local culture can create additional barriers and inhibit the community in fully embracing or owning the healing and recovery process. Thus, in addition to adaptations of more contemporary mental health treatment methods, it is important to enlist vital traditional resources of the society, for instance, its cultural and spiritual healing and recovery practices. Framing the trauma and loss within this context, and providing services tailored to and within it, are essential to achieving and sustaining recovery, resilience, and growth beyond the trauma (Wessels & Monteiro, 2001).

To ensure this cultural sensitivity and relevance, we have found it invaluable to enlist local members of the community, including team members, partners, and trainees, as cultural consultants in appropriately assessing symptoms, needs, and priorities, adapting treatment methods, and incorporating traditional elements and practices. These are essential in ensuring that the end result is a system recognized by, grounded in, and belonging to the community in support of its unique identity.

Empowerment of the Community

A fourth influencing factor is whether capacity for recovery is instilled within the affected community. We have found individual and communal trauma and healing to have a reciprocal and perpetuating influence on one another; in fact, in some sense each is embedded in the other to affect either of two outcomes: alleviating trauma to recover to a healthy state of equilibrium and functioning that supports a positive identity at both levels, or prolonging the trauma and having it become more deeply entrenched. One of the central aspects of this relationship is reflected in the natural interdependency on essential resources at each level:

- The individual's reliance on stable communal resources and support, both informally in terms of social relationships, community identity, and belonging, and formally in terms of civil society systems. When these usual stable social and civil resources of family and community deteriorate or are absent, an individual's likelihood of adequate healing and recovery is severely diminished.
- The community's reliance on a stable resource of skilled and capable members available to maintain civil society systems and social structures, and to reflect the community identity. When there is a scarcity of such competent members, the community's ability to adequately supply support to its members is weakened, or in extreme conditions essentially absent, with the result that the community as a whole risks further decline.

As a result, we have found it necessary to concentrate efforts on addressing recovery at both levels simultaneously.

An underlying principle in this process is employing the human resources of the community itself. It must be empowered with the means needed to resume its central role as the most effective and visible provider of overall well-being for the members of the community. Local capacity-building is particularly indispensable in regions of conflict where service structures, skill resources, and material resources are lacking. In these circumstances, directing aid toward individual and social healing, while actively investing in the local human service system to develop a growing pool of skilled community members, can promote a fuller and more sustainable recovery and post-traumatic growth at every level of society. Benefiting from the same dynamic reciprocal relationship we regularly observe between the individual and communal experience, the deeply powerful symbolism of a community healing itself is vital to regaining the sense of security, esteem, dignity, strength, and balance—with the outside world and within itself—that is threatened and undermined by the trauma experience.

As a result, an effective response to these factors requires using an integrated, whole-person approach for attending to the multiple nature of the refugee experience, as well as the psychosocial–biological–spiritual nature of the severe trauma experience within the local cultural context. At the same time, it is necessary to equip members of the community with varying degrees of practical knowledge, skills, and experience needed to become a self-help community in support of a competent and wholesome community identity.

In sum, focusing assistance on all four key factors of the community-wide trauma experience allows for more successfully endorsing and supporting the healthy internal resources of individuals and their community to strengthen and promote positive transformation in the face of adversity and momentous change.

THE CATASTROPHIC TRAUMA RECOVERY (CTR) MODEL

The Example of Kuwait

Immediately after the withdrawal of Iraqi troops following their invasion of Kuwait in January 1991, a doctor in the main Kuwait City hospital was interviewed on the radio. As the reporter was focused on physical destruction at the ransacked hospital, he asked the doctor to detail what immediate aid they needed from other countries, prompting him with a list of such items as medicine and specialized medical equipment; however, the doctor stopped him short, saying, "We don't need equipment or medicine. We can buy and replace all that quickly and easily. We need therapists." He went on to say, "We have many thousands of people who are emotionally traumatized, and we just don't have the capacity here to help them."

> The pervasive sense of helplessness and threat experienced by most of the population due to the violence and arbitrary nature of the repression used by the Iraqi troops was the contributing factor to the high levels of distress. Unlike many populations that have experienced time-limited events, such as natural disasters, this population was subjected to seven months of traumatic stress. (Eskedal & Behbehani, 1997, p. 142)

At the time, Kuwait had one clinically trained mental health therapist in the country, Dr. Jaafar Mohammad Behbehani, who had coincidentally interned under me, CBI's director, in the mid-1970s in Kalamazoo, Michigan.

The radio interview caught my ear. Unaware of whether Behbehani had returned to Kuwait after obtaining his PhD in England, I contacted the Free Kuwait office in Washington, D.C., to ask what help I could offer. The office was in the process of being dismantled, with the staff returning to Kuwait, but the office director passionately asked for assistance in securing mental health treatment for the massive number of traumatized citizens, among whom were his close family members.

In addition to providing cultural orientation to U.S. therapists planning to travel to Kuwait for brief missions in the weeks and months that followed, I began searching for professional mental health contacts in Kuwait with whom I might communicate regarding conditions on the ground. Through this search, I was eventually reconnected with Behbehani, who, after practicing in London and leading the Association for Free Kuwait there, had moved back to Kuwait City to assist his country. In our phone conversation, Jafaar indicated that, as the only trained therapist in the country, he had been spending his time literally living at the hospital attempting to treat as many victims as possible, while working to train a few MA-level psychology academics on hand in basic treatment methods to assist him. He sounded much sadder than the perpetually cheerful young intern from years before and uncertain about the prospects for the future of his society. Our call ended with my promise to actively pursue support for his efforts. In the ensuing years, CBI solicited assistance from within its international mental health network and regularly referred treatment professionals, organizations, and training resources to Behbehani and his colleagues.

Although there had been assessments of widespread trauma that included concerns about immediate and long-term implications for the society, our search for existing mental health treatment programs by large international professional, humanitarian, or government systems, appropriate and adequate enough to address trauma healing at this large scale, unfortunately failed to find any to which we might direct our colleagues in Kuwait. Instead, we found that the standard approach to addressing such massive needs continued to be furnishing temporary visiting therapists from outside the region, using predominantly Western models and methods limited to treatment at the individual, family, and small group levels, rather than following a more culturally appropriate, multidimensional, and integrated continuum from the individual to the communal experience.

For his part, Behbehani remained in Kuwait to devote himself to developing the local mental health service system. He went on to become one of the pivotal contributors to the development of contemporary Kuwaiti psychology, an expert on PTSD, and a revered teaching mentor to a new generation of mental health professionals in his country prior to his death in 2009.

The Example of the Balkans

In 1992, CBI and its Russian partner, HARMONY Institute, established the Annual International Conference on Conflict Resolution (ICR) in St. Petersburg, Russia. In the 15 years it was held, communal and transgenerational trauma increasingly emerged as frequent themes among participants and in the program. In the late 1990s, near the end of the recent Balkan wars, CBI and HARMONY began bringing representatives of NGO relief and conflict resolution organizations from Kosovo, Serbia, Bosnia, Albania, and Croatia to the ICR conference to take part in a series of special roundtables on the impact of wars on their societies. The first such roundtable occurred, with tensions rising, on the afternoon the Chinese compound in Belgrade was bombed.

Aside from any differences in perspective among roundtable members on the causes of the conflict, the group reached a central and unanimous agreement on the devastating impact of pervasive psychoemotional trauma experienced at every level throughout their societies due to war, the immediate and urgent need for therapy, and the lack of a viable mental health service infrastructure in the region to address the massive need. A second point of agreement was concern that the most current trauma was tapping into past unhealed communal wounds and victim identities dating back generations and even centuries, along with their fear of what this meant for the future potential of their societies for continued and perpetual violence as the single greatest threat to peace and reconciliation in the region.

One example of these unresolved communal traumas embedded in a transgenerational narrative was revealed by a Serbian participant, who, although committed to joining a highly interactive peace conference with members from opposing countries, shared his struggles with his mixed feelings, which offered a window into a cultural victim identity used to fuel and justify much of the inhumane treatment of the Muslim populations in Bosnia and Kosovo. During a time when Serbia was being heavily criticized internationally because of its army's genocidal policies and tactics against civilians, within the Serbian narrative this criticism was felt to be unfair and unjust, particularly coming from their fellow "Christian brothers and sisters" in Europe. The ethnic narrative of the Serbs was that the majority of their male youth had been slaughtered on Kosovo field hundreds of years earlier, on a day commemorated as St. Vitus Day, in a devastating battle where they had acted as a human shield, attempting to stop invading Muslim Ottomans from sweeping into Christian Europe from the East. As a result, their society had been overrun and subjugated for generations.

The Serbian victim story insisted that this profound sacrifice, on a site they called the Field of Blackbirds and considered hallowed ground, had slowed the invaders long enough for Europe to prepare to prevent what they believed would have been the fall of Christian Europe. Although other major geopolitical factors were also in play at the time, the chosen Serbian cultural story, embedded with the trauma, said that it was their sacrifice alone that had saved Europe. Now, centuries later, while being viewed by most of the world as the perpetrator of violence against civilians, a society looking through the lens of its own unresolved transgenerational wounds perceived itself as again fighting the descendants of those Muslim invaders, to drive them out of Bosnia and Kosovo and seek just revenge for their past martyrdom, even as it created new victims and communal wounds, as it contributed to a cycle of violence, trauma, and more violence.

There are many such examples in history, pointing to the implications of profound, unhealed psychoemotional wounding and loss at the communal level, and the toxic energy of even centuries-old transgenerational trauma in fueling future suffering, fear, hostility, and violence—both within and between communities—that further underscore the crucial need for developing effective models and methods for treating at this societal level.

Since CBI and HARMONY are NGOs founded and operated by psychologists, we were asked by these Balkan participants for our help in securing treatment for their communities. Again, as we had experienced with Kuwait several years earlier, we found assessments by large international humanitarian aid systems indicating widespread trauma throughout the Balkans, along with concerns about immediate and long-term implications for these societies; however, as before, our search for existing treatment programs oriented toward and adequate to address trauma at this massive societal level found none. In considering how to respond to these requests, we realized that attempting to drop into the region temporarily to provide traditional direct therapy for hundreds of thousands of people was unrealistic; moreover, it could be only minimally effective at best, even for the largest international aid organizations, let alone grassroots NGOs with limited resources and staff capacity.

In the face of such challenges, it was determined that a different approach was called for, one that NGOs like ours could, in fact, implement successfully. Rather than have a limited number of outside organizations supplying short-term treatment, the idea was instead to focus fully on building local capacity for treatment by instilling the requisite skills and service delivery templates within the impacted community itself; to enable it to become the primary provider of its own healing and recovery—a service that could grow faster, reach more people, and be more permanently sustained.

We began this process by providing trauma treatment skills training to raise the skill level of key local stakeholders already working to aid their communities. Each year, health care professionals and aid workers from regions of conflict and violence, primarily including the Balkans, the Caucasus, and the Middle East, were brought to St. Petersburg for a six-day working conference, which focused on exploring a deeper understanding of individual and communal trauma. They then remained for several days after the event to receive intensive training. Although progress was being made in increasing the amount and quality of treatment services in their communities, as we operated these trainings it was also increasingly apparent that the ratio between the slowly growing pool of trained service providers and the massive, more quickly growing need in their communities severely limited what could be achieved. We understood that, if trauma permeated every level of a society, healing capacity needed to be present at every level as well.

Further expanding on the idea of local capacity-building, then, meant finding ways of tapping into and enlisting the human resources of the entire community, and promoting a continuum of internal healing practices and resources at multiple levels across the society—extending from public education, self-help, and mutual support to highly skilled therapy—as a way to promote creating an empowered self-help community. The approach also needed to be oriented toward the local cultural context and identity, including incorporating traditional healing and recovery customs and being open to ongoing cultural adaptation, so that it would be recognized and owned by the community to ensure the greatest acceptance, integration, effectiveness, and sustainability of the treatment practices. Thus, the perspective on treatment, healing, and resilience-building was widened to include a spectrum of strengths and skills that could be woven into the community at various levels, to contribute to overall individual and communal wellness.

To help in organizing and framing the different aspects of this concept, I first created a structural outline as a guide for further extension and improvement. This was subsequently developed into the Catastrophic Trauma Recovery (CTR) Model, as an integrated, whole-person training and treatment approach to addressing large-scale, community-wide trauma and loss due to catastrophic occurrences, particularly in regions where the local human service infrastructure was absent, underdeveloped, or compromised, and where skills and hard resources were scarce.

The model's central principles are local capacity-building, cultural adaptation, and community empowerment through becoming the predominant source of its own repair. It uses both proven skills and cultural strengths, seen as essential to regaining, supporting, and maintaining a confident, positive, and resilient community identity.

THE CTR MODEL IS BASED ON A PYRAMID STRUCTURE

The pyramid structure has the following purposes:

- Establishing a broad foundation within the general public of mental health education, along with self-help and peer-support skills for the layperson, to reach and assist the most people, help bolster mutual support, and reduce mental health stigmas in the immediate short term.
- Supporting community service providers, for example, medical practitioners, teachers, and clergy, with basic intervention skills and knowledge of trauma-related symptoms and behaviors, to help them better understand, respond to, and support those they encounter who exhibit these attributes.

- Progressively building an expanding number of increasingly skilled paraprofessionals and professionals with expertise in psychosocial treatment and recovery services in the long term.
- Establishing pilot community-based psychosocial service projects to demonstrate service delivery templates that can be successful in communities where the mental health service system is underdeveloped and where skills and hard resources are scarce.

Rather than being limited to any one particular specialized treatment method, CTR promotes an interdisciplinary, eclectic, and culturally adaptive approach, employing a variety of therapeutic practices and modalities tailored to the needs and character of the individuals and the community, addressing both psychoemotional–biological–spiritual needs and interrelated concrete socioeconomic needs required to achieve full day-to-day stability and recovery. It also incorporates traditional aspects of the culture, as it supports and promotes strategic collaboration with indigenous stakeholders and human services to benefit from group strengths and promote the system being fully owned by the community.

Its features include the following:

- Public mental health education, to increase mental health awareness and promote good health practices in support of community well-being.
- Self-help, coping, and personal development skills, instilled in members of the community to increase capacity for self-care and mutual emotional support
- Socio-economic-educational support and stabilization.
- Communal healing and resilience-building in the form of events and activities that employ and incorporate traditional, spiritual, and newly created healing and renewal rituals and ceremonies; build and reinforce cultural narratives of recovery, resilience, solidarity, and communal esteem; and tap into the internal community resources to develop an empowered, self-help identity.
- Trauma-informed community services that support local social service providers (medical practitioners, clergy and spiritual leaders, teachers, law enforcement, etc.) by equipping them with basic psychosocial orientation and intervention skills to more effectively identify, engage with, and assist individuals exhibiting behavioral and emotional trauma symptoms, and assess them for referral to more in-depth treatment where indicated.
- Community intervention, mediation, and victim advocacy to model and nurture community acceptance and build capacity for support of victims, particularly victims of rape and sexual abuse, who often face a secondary trauma of blame and rejection.

- Psychosocial training and direct treatment services to invest in the local human service and educational systems to create a regularly expanding number of treatment personnel by providing professional and paraprofessional certified skills training, in partnership with local universities, professional institutes and associations, social service and community organizations, and government bodies. Also to use trainees in establishing and operating community-based direct service programs or supporting existing programs to provide crisis intervention and stabilization services (site-based, phone, and outreach), and trauma-informed therapy for individuals, families, and groups, in the form of a broad spectrum of interdisciplinary and culturally adapted approaches and methods for treating trauma and other mental health issues.
- Support and sustaining of local psychosocial service providers and services, including self-care and burnout prevention, training of trainers, service program design, development, and implementation based on strategic collaboration, and ongoing consultation and mentoring support.

Since the CTR model was first developed, community-based, local capacity-building training and treatment programs based on it have been conducted through our work in various regions where local services and skill resources are limited. The most current example is the certified SHC training and treatment program operated by CBI and the International Humanistic Psychology Association (IHPA) in Jordan since 2012, to address the Syrian refugee crisis. In recent years, this partnership has expanded to include Michigan State University's Department of Psychiatry, as well as all Jordanian medical schools, the Queen Rania Center, the International Federation of Medical Student Associations–Jordan (IFMSA-J), and local human service NGOs.

THE SOCIAL HEALTH CARE (SHC) TRAINING AND TREATMENT PROGRAM

Today we are witnessing yet another immense humanitarian crisis with Syrian refugees scattered throughout the Middle East and increasingly worldwide. Widespread and devastating psychoemotional wounds once again pose a profound and lasting threat to the long-term stability and well-being of an entire society, as well as to the region of which they are a part, underscoring the imperative for developing new models and methods in treating trauma at this scale.

In addition to the suffering of the Syrian population itself, countries in a part of the world already challenged by severely limited resources and facing the sudden and catastrophic needs of massive numbers of refugees pouring

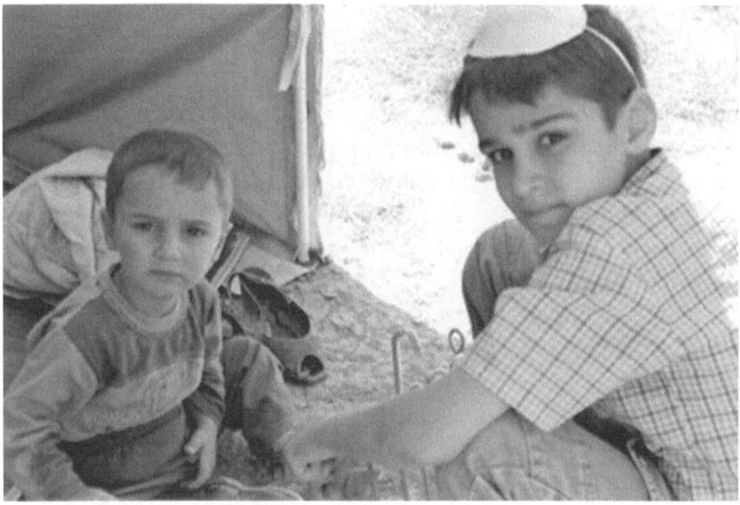

Figure 11.2. Brothers at CBI field clinic. Zaatari Refugee Camp, Jordan.

across their borders seeking safety from the conflict are increasingly overwhelmed. This is particularly the experience of Jordan, a poor country with an enormous unemployment rate, which for almost three-quarters of a century has struggled with accommodating the needs of a steady influx of refugees fleeing conflict and turmoil from countries on its borders (Chatelard, 2010). It is here that CBI has been applying the CTR Model in developing and conducting a tailored humanitarian aid program to address the Syrian refugee crisis.

The Syrian civil war, which at the time of this writing has been raging for almost eight years, has seen an even greater surge in refugees entering the country and further straining the limits of its ability to care for their most basic needs while also attempting to care for its own population. As millions of Syrians move away to escape the danger and turmoil, many arrive in Jordan and surrounding countries suffering from profound and debilitating psychoemotional trauma (Hadid, 2016).

At the same time, the mental health service system in Jordan and the region in general is seriously underdeveloped and ill-equipped to meet the demands. Other than in the case of a small portion of wealthy citizens able to access the tiny pool of trained professional therapists in the country, mental health treatment beyond receiving medication or being confined to hospitals for the most extreme at-risk cases is essentially nonexistent for the Jordanian population, and particularly so for refugees (International Medical Corps, 2017).

In our meetings with the administrations of all Jordanian universities, it was confirmed that, at the root of this deficit in growing an adequate local mental health service system, is a lack of practical academic or professional mental health training programs within the country. Historically, students in mental health disciplines looking for practical skills training have been required to seek internships outside of Jordan and the region. Of the small number who are accepted and have the financial means to take advantage of these opportunities, very few ever return to benefit their home society. The result has been a continual talent drain, as the society's need for these services only multiplies.

In response to one of the most recent crises in the Middle East, CBI and IHPA established the SHC program in 2012—an integrated, certified training and pilot service initiative using a psychosocial–biological–spiritual approach. It focuses on individual and social healing, sustainable recovery, and self-determination, while actively investing in the local human service and educational systems.

In keeping with the CTR Model, the emphasis is on innovative and local capacity-building approaches to using the internal human and sociocultural resources of the community, and promoting the individual and communal narratives and identities of resilient, empowered survivors and psychosocial growth. It teaches a humanistic, holistic, and interdisciplinary orientation, with a strong focus on developing an eclectic repertoire of treatment methods adapted to the local culture.

The two features of the SHC program are training and treatment.

Training

This process involves instilling restorative resources within the community by equipping its members at every level with varying degrees of practical knowledge, skills, and experience. These range from self-help to in-depth psychosocial therapy to promote a self-healing community.

Another aspect is investing in the local human service and educational systems through providing certified training for professionals in mental health-related disciplines, in partnership with local universities. Training is also provided for paraprofessionals, humanitarian aid workers, and civil society service providers working with refugees and vulnerable populations.

To the Public and Service Recipient Community

- Public mental health education. Public education is offered to service recipients and the general public on mental health issues and symptoms, to reduce stigma, increase mental health understanding and knowledge of available treatment resources, and promote good health practices.

- Self-help, coping, and personal development skills training to service recipients. These are offered to increase the ability for self-care in management of stress, mood, and behavior to build emotional stability, self-control, confidence, and self-esteem, and increase the ability to offer mutual emotional support and reassurance to family, neighbors, and other community members using learned self-care and supportive listening skills.

To Local Service Providers Working with Refugees and Vulnerable Populations

The certified professional and paraprofessional training program uses a variety of interdisciplinary therapeutic approaches, methods, and techniques, adapted to the local culture, for treating trauma and other mental health issues. Examples include the following:

- psychosocial assessment and treatment planning
- brief therapeutic intervention methods and strategies
- expressive arts therapies
- Somatic therapies
- faith and spiritual-based therapies
- in-depth, longer-term psychotherapies
- medication where indicated for symptom relief in support of therapy

Targeted trainees include local students; NGO staff; social and human service providers; and relief workers in relevant fields, including psychology, psychiatry, social work, counseling, medicine, teaching, and religion. Priority is given to members of the refugee community, those working with refugees and other vulnerable at-risk populations, and those who are in positions to model and teach skills to others.

Components of training to service providers include the following:

1. Community-Based Psychosocial Skills Training Program. This provides a certified progressive training and practice in psychosocial support and treatment skills generally open to local trainees. Both professional and paraprofessional service providers are prepared to deliver a range of direct treatment services, from coping skills and crisis intervention and stabilization, to more advanced psychosocial treatments. Trainees include university students and faculty, local humanitarian aid NGO staff, nurses, aid workers, teachers, and other human service workers.
2. Psychosocial Specialty Training (PST) for medical students and practitioners. A landmark, fully certified professional training and field experience program in psychosocial assessment and treatment skills, incorporated into the formal medical school academic programs for all

fifth- and sixth-year medical students in Jordan. The certified training is provided in partnership with the five Jordanian medical schools, Michigan State University's Department of Psychiatry, and IFMSA-J. It offers two levels:

- Preparing medical doctors of all specialties with essential skills that they can incorporate into their general medical practice.
- Providing longer-term, more in-depth training and experience to medical students wishing to specialize in psychiatry, leading to opportunities for additional advanced training with Michigan State's Department of Psychiatry in preparation for future psychiatric internships.

The program's humanistic psychology and interdisciplinary team orientation, strong focus on developing an eclectic skill set, and emphasis on therapy are geared toward preparing psychiatrists to play key roles within an interdisciplinary community mental-health team model.

3. Certified Diploma in Clinical Social Work. This is a university-based certified practical diploma program preparing social work students in Jordan with training and field experience in practical social work, enabling them to administer direct services to at-risk and unserved populations. The program is conducted by CBI and certified in partnership with Yarmouk University, the Queen Rania Center for Jordanian Studies and Community Service, and Michigan State University.
4. Psychosocial Training for Clergy and Religious Teachers. First developed by Michigan State University's Department of Psychiatry, this program is administered by CBI and IHPA, in partnership with Michigan State University. This interreligious faith-based training component is conducted specifically for religious leaders, students, and teachers, focusing on psychoemotional symptoms and behaviors, basic responses, and supportive counseling to assist those exhibiting symptoms. Trainees learn when referral to a professional therapist is indicated and also how to handle unique situations and stresses clergy and religious teachers encounter with many who are suffering from mental health difficulties. The training component is conducted in partnership with Yarmouk University's Department of Religion.
5. Training of Trainers. This part of the program aims to develop and support a local pool of expert trainers and mentors, through advanced certified training and supervised experience in teaching and supervision skills for those completing the SHC training program at a high level of proficiency.

6. Growth, support, and sustaining of local service providers and community services.

- Self-care and burnout prevention for service providers to manage the anticipated stress and high potential for burnout. It includes stress management skills training and peer support and supervision groups for ongoing support and consultation.
- Service program development and innovation. This involves modeling and demonstrating creative innovations in designing, implementing, scaling up, and replicating pilot service programs; the emphasis is on working with scarce resources and promoting a model of strategic collaboration and partnership to build additional capacity for providing and quickly expanding services on a continuing basis.
- Ongoing consultation and mentoring support by clinical training faculty.
- Ongoing access to CBI and university online training resource libraries, including multimedia professional materials and modules (audio and video programs, taped training sessions, web-based interactive training programs, written manuals and program materials, assessment tools, journals, etc.).

Proposed future development involves the following programs:

1. Practical MA in community mental health treatment: a two-year certified practical MA in community mental health treatment, in partnership with Jordanian universities and Michigan State University.
2. Biregional cross-training for psychosocial services to refugees: A biregional collaboration between professional groups in Jordan and countries hosting Middle Eastern refugees to share culturally adapted psychosocial treatment services and cultural competency training.

Treatment

Psychosocial treatment activities provide the following:

- Direct treatment, along with coping and personal development skills training for refugees and vulnerable populations.
- Field experience opportunities for trainers/therapists to demonstrate and model methods and for trainees to practice learned skills in the field, under supervision.
- Practical pilot service projects to demonstrate designing, implementing, scaling up, replicating, and sustaining holistic, community mental health services that local NGOs and trainees are prepared to operate.

Current treatment components are as follows:

- Disaster Health Care Field Clinics, which provide short-term intensive field clinics offering direct psychosocial and medical screening and treatment services to refugee children and their families.
- Community-Based Pilot Service Projects, created in cooperation with local SHC team members and trainees and NGO partners, who are prepared for operating, further developing, and sustaining them on an ongoing basis. The services and activities that they offer address multiple interrelated need areas essential to recovery and long-term stability, and are designed to be scalable, portable, and replicated. Service recipients and local site staff are also provided with English-language lessons to increase efficiency in communicating with visiting clinical team members and accessing English language–based services and resources.

Service project examples include the following:

1. Residential Service Center. A secure, supportive living environment housing 40 families exclusively made up of Syrian refugee widows and their children, where recovery activities are provided to adult and child residents, including a variety of psychosocial treatment services, medical health screening, support groups, coping and personal development skills training, vocational and educational skills support to prepare heads of household for independence, and recreational and resilience-building activities. Residential management staff are offered basic support and intervention skills training to increase their ability to support residents.
2. Women's Safe Spaces. Dedicated spaces in partnering day-service centers where vulnerable refugee women and girls can gather to feel secure in receiving a variety of support services, for example, psychosocial counseling support, support groups, coping and personal development skills training, parenting skills, education and materials on women's health issues, medical health screening, support for pregnant women and new mothers, basic personal needs, educational and vocational skills support, exercise, crafts and creative activities, and a mutual support system to reduce stress and exploitation, while promoting self-esteem, resilience, and empowerment.
3. Youth and Community Resilience-Building. An activities program to bolster and nourish internal resources and the capacity of individuals and the community for recreation; peer interaction that promotes positive values and nonviolent communication; appreciation for communal traditions; child protection; and joy for refugee children, their families, and community. Examples include nature excursions; recrea-

tional activities; community social and cultural events; and teaching self-help skills, mutual support, and teamwork using games, cooperative sports, and expressive arts.

4. Trauma-Informed Educational Recovery Project. This project teaches coping and resilience-building, which includes stress management, self-soothing, nonviolent communication, and conflict resolution skills training for students, while promoting the incorporation of this material into the regular school curriculum to become a "trauma-informed school." Basic training for schoolteachers and administrators is provided in identifying, understanding, and being sensitive to trauma symptoms, as well as learning basic supportive responses to students and their parents. It provides student and school support, through assisting students and schools for refugees in obtaining needed school tuition, materials, and supplies to recover from educational deficits and maintain access to schooling. It also provides English as a second language (ESL) training to allow students and teachers access to English-based educational resource materials and online classes, and to communicate more effectively with English-based humanitarian aid services.
5. Socioeconomic Empowerment Project. This project equips vulnerable Syrian refugee women, widows, and adolescent heads of household with the means to care for the economic, health, and security needs of their families, increasing their self-sufficiency, self-confidence, and dignity, while reducing exploitation. Services include training in coping and personal development skills, marketable vocational skills, employment preparation, and small business/cottage industry start-up mentoring.

PROFESSIONAL DEVELOPMENT, RESEARCH, AND COALITION BUILDING

To promote and support the qualities of collaboration, shared knowledge, and shared experience among psychosocial professionals, and to provide further professional learning for our trainees, CBI regularly conducts and integrates relevant activities. These are designed to place issues of individual and communal trauma on the public table for awareness raising and mutual exploration through topical training conferences, research activities, and related publications. Included in the research aspect is the study of the SHC program and its various components. These activities are as follows:

- The Annual International Conference on Transgenerational Trauma (TT). CBI has a history of organizing more than 50 international professional conferences on social healing and conflict transformation since 1992, in various countries, particularly in developing societies in regions of conflict. Its most recent conference series is the Annual International Conference on Transgenerational Trauma, held each fall in Jordan. The TT Conference is an international working conference that brings together practitioners, trainers, and researchers from throughout the world to: share practical skills, theory, and research; develop new culturally adaptable models and methods for better addressing large scale communal and transgenerational trauma; and formulate recommendations and guidelines for communities and public policymakers. CBI's conferences are highly interactive and action-oriented, promoting skills acquisition and practical outcomes and applications. The SHC program grew out of these conferences; as a result, as a part of their SHC program, trainees participate in them to gain additional skills through presenters' workshops.

- Transgenerational Trauma Research Network. This is a developing collaborative network promoting concerted interdisciplinary and cross-cultural study of the dimensions, dynamics, and implications of communal and transgenerational trauma, and the development of practical approaches to large-scale trauma.
- *Journal of Communal and Transgenerational Trauma.* This is a new virtual international professional journal being established in support of the TT Conference and research network. It is a multimedia publication geared to both professionals and the lay public.

Additional Applications for Refugees Beyond Jordan

Increasingly, CBI is offering consultation, training, and service models designed to help meet the unique needs of organizations within host communities in countries outside of the regions that are currently receiving refugees. Examples of assistance include working with war trauma; building cultural competency; and establishing trauma-informed educational and cultural transition programs to assist refugee students arriving with limited formal schooling, local language skills, and cultural orientation.

CONCLUSION

The CTR Model, and the SHC program based on it, is one example of a whole-person, cross-cultural approach to addressing the complex dynamics of catastrophic trauma at the individual and communal levels. It is an evolving model, and, in the case of its application in Jordan, it is designed to take on the local cultural character increasingly throughout time, as it develops into a uniquely Jordanian version.

Linked to the principles of local capacity-building and cultural adaptation for social healing, which are at the center of the model, is an emphasis on and commitment to strategic collaboration with other like-purposed organizations, particularly including local colleagues, NGOs, and institutions in the impacted community. CBI and IHPA work closely with these colleagues and organizations in developing, adapting, and implementing these initiatives within their home society. As we contribute our skill resources and supporting networks, we also rely on local partners to assist us with on-site staffing, providing and coordinating training and service site logistics, identifying and enlisting trainees, and helping to network with other organizations and government entities.

Partnering with and mutually supporting local humanitarian service organizations and colleagues, as well as vital institutions like universities, are fundamental to our historical philosophy and essential to the success of our efforts in various regions for nearly three decades.

Given this history, our view during this same period has been that, in the face of massive human suffering and hardship—most in regions of the world where trauma has become systemic and humanitarian aid systems and resources are scarce—any approach to healing trauma at the large scale requires a commitment to such a model of cooperation, collaboration, and mutual support. The sheer size of catastrophic humanitarian crises increasingly seen throughout the world is ill-served by stand-alone initiatives working in isolation, or at times even in competition with others, that serve to generate gaps, duplication, wasted resources, and missed opportunities.

There are now more than 68 million people in the world being driven from their homes, with almost 26 million refugees fleeing for their lives from armed conflict and violence. Of these, more than 16 million fled in 2017 alone, at an increasing rate of more than one person uprooted every two seconds (UNHCR, 2018). Confronted with this unprecedented mass displacement, it is painfully evident to anyone directly working in these settings that even the largest organizations attempting to operate on their own are continually falling behind, as the crisis only grows. We see the lack of adequate coordination and cooperation by humanitarian aid organizations as one of the major challenges to meeting the needs of traumatized communities—a challenge that calls for new thinking and commitment to a new model of strategic collaboration.

Although pervasive communal trauma, and the prospect of transgenerational trauma to which it can lead, poses significant and mounting challenges to the field of mental health globally, through shared knowledge and concerted efforts these challenges can be increasingly and effectively addressed, if we act together. The most practical and responsible path with the most promise is through a willingness to engage and collaborate with all stakeholders, learning from our mutual efforts to complement, support, and build on one another's work, where truly effective organizations provide the essential pieces of a larger humanitarian assistance puzzle that combines to reach further, faster, and accomplish more in service to those in desperate need.

REFERENCES

Butler, A., Panzer, A., & Goldfrank, L. (eds.) (2003). *Preparing for the psychological consequences of terrorism: A public health strategy*. Washington, DC: National Academies Press.

Chatelard, Geraldine. (2010, August 31). Jordan: A refugee haven. *Migration Policy Institute*. Retrieved from https://www.migrationpolicy.org/article/jordan-refugee-haven.

Davis, R., Pinderhughes, H., & Williams, M. (2016, February). Adverse community experiences and resilience: A framework for addressing and preventing community trauma. *Prevention Institute*. Retrieved fromhttps://www.preventioninstitute.org/publications/adverse-community-experiences-and-resilience-framework-addressing-and-preventing.

Eskedal, G., & Behbehani, J. (1997, Spring). Kuwait connection: An international training experience. *McGill Journal of Education*, *32*(2), 139–48.

Hadid, Farah Al. (2016, February 20). Mental health of Syrian refugees in Jordan. *Yale Global Health Review*. Retrieved from https://yaleglobalhealthreview.com/2016/02/20/mental-health-of-syrian-refugees-in-jordan/.

International Medical Corps. (2017, February 5). *Assessment report: Understanding the mental health and psychosocial needs, and service utilization of Syrian refugees and Jordanian nationals*. Retrieved from https://reliefweb.int/sites/reliefweb.int/files/resources/JordanAssessmentReport-UnderstandingtheMentalHealthandPsychosocialNeedsand ServiceUtilizationofSyrianRefugeesandJordanianNationals.pdf.

Milroy, H., & Zubrick, S. R. (2005). *The Western Australian Aboriginal Child Health Survey: The social and emotional well-being of aboriginal children and young people*. Perth, Australia: Curtin University.

Olweean, S. (2002). Psychological concepts of the "other": Embracing the compass of the self. In C. Stout (ed.), *The psychology of terrorism: A public understanding* (pp. 113–28). Westport, CT: Praeger.

Olweean, S. (2003). When society is the victim: Catastrophic trauma recovery. In S. Krippner & T. McIntyre (eds.), *The psychological impact of war trauma on civilians: An international perspective* (pp. 271–76). Westport, CT: Praeger.

Silove, D., Ventevogel, P., & Rees, S. (2017, June). The contemporary refugee crisis: An overview of mental health challenges. *World Psychiatry*, *16*(2), 130–39. doi: 10.1002/wps.20438.

UNHCR. (2018, May 15). Global trends report. Retrieved fromhttps://www.unhcr.org/globaltrends2017/.

Volkan, V. (1998). *Bloodlines: From ethnic pride to ethnic terrorism*. Boulder, CO: Westview Press.

Wessels, M., & Monteiro, C. (2001). Psychosocial intervention and postwar reconstruction in Angola: Interweaving Western and traditional approaches. In D. J. Christie, R. V. Wagner, & D. A. Winter (eds.), *Peace, conflict, and violence: Peace psychology for the 21st century* (pp. 262–76). Englewood Cliffs, NJ: Prentice-Hall.

Wessels, M., & Monteiro, C. (2003). Healing, social integration, and community mobilization for war-affected children: A view from Angola. In S. Krippner & T. McIntyre (eds.), *The psychological impact of war trauma on civilians: An international perspective* (pp. 179–91). Westport, CT: Praeger.

IV

Future of Integrative Care for the Traumatized

Chapter Twelve

Promoting Caregiver Satisfaction and Regeneration

Eleanor Pardess

This chapter presents a multimodal model for preventing compassion fatigue and promoting caregiver satisfaction and regeneration. Initially developed by the Israel Crisis Management SELAH (a Hebrew word meaning "a rock to lean upon"), this model integrates various modalities, including nature-based activities, mindfulness practices, and intermodal expressive arts. Rather than focusing exclusively on stress management, the model aims to provide a secure base for exploration and growth. It uses metaphors to open space for reflection and to convey ideas and feelings that often cannot easily be put into words (Kopp, 1995).

The focus of the chapter is on the potential of nature-based workshops, one of the components of the SELAH model. The workshops are combined with mindfulness practices and expressive modalities, as part of a whole-person approach (Serlin, 2007; Serlin & Cannon, 2004; Serlin & Hansen, 2015). They are integrated into the training and support programs for caregivers that provide emergency first aid and long-term support in the aftermath of trauma. The illustrations and research findings highlight the potential power of these programs to prevent burnout and promote compassion satisfaction and regeneration.

UNDERSTANDING COMPASSION FATIGUE

Caregiver burnout and compassion fatigue are currently receiving significant attention from health care practitioners (Cocker & Joss, 2016). *Compassion fatigue* refers to the emotional impact of working with people involved in traumatizing life events, for example, terrorist attacks, war, torture, family violence, criminal assault, or sexual violation. The demanding nature of this work and the intense exposure to human suffering can lead to what has been called secondary or vicarious traumatization. Caregivers are subject to risks ranging from emotional exhaustion, heightened anxiety, and nightmares and other sleep disturbances, to secondary traumatization marked by the full range of PTSD (Figley, 1995, 2002).

Compassion fatigue, which is a combination of burnout and traumatization, engenders significant costs for trauma workers and the quality of care they provide (Figley, 2002; McCann & Pearlman, 1990). The profound impact on personal well-being and professional function can manifest itself across psychological, cognitive, and interpersonal domains. Symptoms of compassion fatigue are similar to the three classic features of PTSD: 1) hyperarousal, disturbed sleep, irritability, and hypervigilance; 2) intrusive thoughts and worries, and 3) avoidance, as in "not wanting to go there again" and the desire to avoid thoughts, feelings, and conversations associated with the care recipient's pain and suffering (Figley, 2002; Rothschild, 2006).

The effects of compassion fatigue may worsen throughout time, compromising caregivers' ability to interact in positive and helpful ways with traumatized individuals and their families (Craig & Sprang, 2010). Caregivers who do not receive adequate support may soon find their emotional resources depleted (Figley, 2002; Vachon, 2015).

The multifaceted nature of the caregiver experience calls for an integrative perspective. Caregivers, who navigate situations of severe distress, do this challenging work while confronting the intense emotions of the traumatized and their families. To reduce this risk of compassion fatigue, ongoing support is imperative to conserve and strengthen the caregivers' inner resources to meet the demands they face (Pardess, 2005; Pearlman & Caringi, 2009; Sodeke-Gregson, Holttum, & Billings, 2013).

The whole-person approach is a particularly relevant framework for building such resourcefulness due to its integration of cutting-edge practices in a bio–psycho–spiritual model supporting resilience and growth. It represents a paradigm shift from an illness model to a growth-oriented model. Extensive research has been conducted on programs for "helping the helper," but the current literature has focused almost exclusively on the negative consequences of caregiving (Pardess, 2005) at the expense of exploring the entire spectrum of the caregiving experience (Linley & Joseph, 2007). Witnessing suffering and struggling with adversity, according to the SELAH strength-based model described in this chapter, may lead to the discovery of strengths and the enhancement of life's meaning. This model calls for widening the circles of compassionate care through cultivating presence, emotional regulation, and openness to experience.

One of the unique contributions of this model is the integration of nature-based experiential activities with mindfulness and compassionate mind training. The incorporation of both verbal and nonverbal creative modalities creates a wide spectrum of opportunities for self-expression, enabling caregivers to find their own voice and expand strategies for regaining calm in the face of turbulence. This integrative approach adds a new dimension to conventional "helping the helper" programs by "giving voice" and fostering a sense of belonging among caregivers.

AN INTEGRATIVE MODEL

SELAH, the Israel Crisis Management Center, is a nonprofit organization supporting immigrants coping with traumatic loss due to terrorist attacks and other disasters. The multidisciplinary teams provide immediate on-site emergency practical assistance and emotional support to the bereaved, as well as the wounded and their families, from the initial hours after tragedy strikes, followed by long-term individual and group support.

SELAH's two- and three-day seminars are an integral part of this comprehensive support program. The seminars, which are held in different locations in Israel, are tailored to meet the needs of different target groups, including bereaved parents, widows/widowers, grandparents raising orphaned grandchildren, and children and adolescents coping with the sudden death or severe wounding of a family member. Each of these groups deals with specific themes, but the programs share the common goal of strengthening secure connections, cultivating meaning, and creating a safe space for sharing and bearing witness.

Since isolation is a crucial risk factor in the aftermath of trauma (Neuschul & Page, 2018), breaking through isolation is one of the goals of the SELAH programs. Support from the multidisciplinary teams, in addition to the mutual support of others in the group, is woven together, step by step, to create a "safety net"—a caring community. The caregivers themselves attend the seminars, in addition to having individual and group supervision, and taking part in training programs and workshops (Pardess, 2005).

Measures That May Help Prevent Burnout and Compassion Fatigue

"The expectation that we can be immersed in suffering and loss daily and not be touched by it is as unrealistic as expecting to be able to walk through water without getting wet" (Remen, 1996). What can caregivers do to protect themselves from the stress that "comes with the territory" of trauma work? The following are a number of suggestions that have been offered by caregivers as strategies for mitigating compassion fatigue and promoting regeneration:

- Engage in such self-care behaviors as getting adequate sleep, balanced nutrition, and regular exercise.
- Practice mindfulness, breathing, and visual imagery.
- Engage regularly in pleasurable activities to rejuvenate and restore energy and joy.
- Maintain a good balance between work and family, and developing supportive relationships with family and friends outside of work.
- Find and allow for adequate personal time to grieve losses and process difficult experiences that are evoked in encounters with the traumatized.
- Develop a philosophy of care that cultivates a sense of meaning and purpose.

Professional Development Strategies

- Allow yourself to be moved and challenged by the people you meet and their physical, emotional, and spiritual problems without making them your own; view the encounters with people who you find most difficult as a growth-promoting experience and an opportunity to transcend your boundaries and deepen compassion.
- Recognize that you are not alone in facing the stresses of working with the traumatized.
- Be clear and consistent with yourself and others about your boundaries and personal limit-setting (including taking vacations, learning to say "no," and asking for what you need).
- Connect often with a respectful team that meets regularly and shares a common goal or mission.

Traditionally, self-care strategies have emphasized the value of "good professional boundaries" and effective self-care strategies outside the workplace. These alone, however, can lead to emotional detachment by the caregiver. Over-reliance on strategies of avoidance can result in diminished compassion satisfaction (Pardess et al., 2009). By blending the expressive arts with nature-based activities, the SELAH model offers caregivers tools for the regulation of levels of arousal and validation of their own experience. This expands their ability to take care of personal, familial, and emotional needs, while attending to the needs of care recipients. One of the key messages in the program is, "If your compassion does not include yourself, it is incomplete" (Kornfield, 1994, p. 28).

THE NATURE-BASED WORKSHOPS

Since many of the SELAH caregivers are immigrants from diverse backgrounds, group excursions were planned in the first programs initiated more than 20 years ago, as an opportunity for them to get to know the country. These outings, which were called "Walking the Bible," included visits to places of historical significance. The trips were designed to promote a sense of belonging and provide a wider context and perspective for personal trauma and loss. The more practical applications, based on metaphors from nature, compassionate imagery, and mindfulness practices, were incorporated at a later stage of the development of the program. The nature-based workshops remain one of the components of the caregiver seminars.

The following sequence of experiential activities in each of these workshops was designed to enable a gradual entry and engagement of participants in the process, which unfolds as it goes along. The following is the structure of a typical workshop:

1. Grounding: Grounding is the first step in establishing a safe and secure atmosphere for identifying natural resources.
2. Cultivating presence: Participants are invited to slow down and notice mindfully what bodily sensations come up as they become more present in the "here and now." (For example, "We need to slow down to be present with ourselves and others, and curious enough about what is happening within ourselves.")
3. Mindful walking in nature and guided imagery: The walk takes place along a route preplanned by the staff on the basis of the workshop topic and its participants. While walking, participants are invited to allow their senses to open up to the surroundings—to look, listen, touch, and smell. The experiential activities at the various stations along the way are adjusted to the composition and needs of the specific groups of caregivers, while including a great deal of space for reflection and spontaneous development of topics raised by the participants.
4. Multimodal creative activity: After returning to an indoor setting, participants are invited to follow the lead of the items spread around the room (including materials from nature, newspaper clippings, old calendars, and coloring materials).
5. Reconnecting: In the final phase, participants are invited to share their creations and reflect on the process they experienced during the different parts of the workshop. What did they encounter on the walk that was meaningful for them? To what were their eyes drawn? Discussions may focus on identifying resources that may be taken from the different parts of the workshop and mobilized in challenging encoun-

ters. The workshop closes with a poem composed by the group facilitator, constructed of phrases or sentences selected from the participants' expressions and elaborating on the metaphors offered during the workshop.

The following section describes the use of metaphors and how the nature-based activities are tailored to cultivate mindful presence and nurture the capacity of caregivers to balance between caring for others and caring for themselves.

Harnessing the Power of Metaphors from Nature

The word *metaphor* is Greek in origin, stemming from *meta* (change) and *pherein* (to bear, or to carry). The word *amphora*, which has the same root, refers to an ancient Greek vessel for carrying and storing precious liquids. Metaphors can carry ideas and feelings that cannot be put into words (Kopp, 1995). Using metaphors from nature in group work, combined with mindfulness practices and expressive modalities as part of a whole-person approach, can open up new possibilities for balancing caring for self and others, and building bridges between the past, present, and future.

Understanding natural processes of regeneration and the interconnectedness of the web of life offers a wider perspective that may open new meanings in the encounter with suffering. Awareness of the multiple ways in which life unfolds and interacts with both death and the regenerative processes in nature can help caretakers feel more rooted in humility. Compassion is connected to our willingness to acknowledge the ways in which we are both powerful and vulnerable, and to understand how we are interdependent on one another.

In the immediate aftermath of traumatizing events, caregivers often desperately need support; however, too much exposure can be overwhelming. That is why a nonintrusive, indirect approach, for instance, the use of imagery, is so crucial. Caregivers are invited to share their own unique ways of grounding themselves and engaging inner balance.

For example, in one workshop we discuss the various mechanisms trees use to protect themselves in a fire or the "survival mode" of desert plants. Upon reflecting on such protective strategies as "closing down" or going into "safe mode," caregivers often describe feeling numb as a result of being flooded by overwhelming stress. "It is as if you are a sponge that is completely saturated and has never been wrung out" (Lipsky, 2009, p. 104). Such metaphors are explored and expanded on by group participants, for example, "I would like to cover myself with a layer of wax to protect myself," in the words of a caregiver in one of the seminars held after a difficult period of multiple terrorist attacks.

Caregivers have their own ways of coping, but it is important to help them identify and use them to the best of their ability. Sharing perspectives in a validating atmosphere demonstrates the value of diversity and respect for individual differences. The experiential activities in the workshops offer participants opportunities for resourcing, as well as finding new ways to approach the challenges they face in a proactive, rather than a reactive, way.

The Wounded Healer

The term *wounded healer* was used by Jung (1951), drawing on the image of Chiron, the archetypal wounded healer in Greek mythology. Chiron, who was the wisest of the Centaurs, was wounded in battle by an arrow and became very ill. The resultant anguish set him on a journey of discovery in search of his own cure. Along the way, he discovered his healing powers and ability to alleviate suffering. By helping others, he found a safe haven of healing for himself. Chiron's courage to be in touch with his wound was the key to his special healing powers (Rice, 2011).

Some of the former participants have become SELAH volunteers. Drawing on their personal experience, they offer valuable insights into transforming pain and posttraumatic growth. One of these is Nadia Ganzman of Nazareth Elite, who immigrated to Israel from Belarus in 1991, and then lost her only son, Valery, in Lebanon in 1996. "I felt all alone in Israel," she said.

> My husband and I came to this country because of Valery, because of his love of Israel. I didn't understand how it was possible to go on living—to enjoy life. But then four months after my son fell, a woman came to see me whose only son had fallen three years before. She showed me that I was not alone. She helped me to meet others overcoming the same loss. I realized that I could go on. And little by little, I began living again. I decided I wanted to give back what I received. So now I reach out to bereaved families and bring them the message that they are not alone. I wanted to do so before the training program, but I had no idea how to do so. Everything seemed so futile before the seminar. I felt so blocked that I could not even imagine myself being around people. It is still hard, really hard, for me to make these visits, but I also feel a deeper connection to other people and feel more in touch with myself. It keeps me going.

Anna Krakovich of Haifa, a former English teacher, is an example of a survivor of a terrorist attack who has become a SELAH volunteer. More than 70% of her body was burned in a car bomb explosion in 1994, two years after she immigrated to Israel with her young daughter. She was not expected to live. Said Anna,

> When I opened my eyes in the hospital, I saw a strange woman sitting by me. I was in so much pain that I spent nearly a year there, talking with the wounded.

> I could see that they were glad I didn't have the strength to ask what was uppermost in my mind—where was my daughter Irene? I couldn't remember what had happened, or if Irene had been with me. Without my asking, Ruth Bar-On from SELAH said to me, "Don't worry, Irene is safe." She knew instinctively what my primary concern would be.

Krakovich spent 11 months in the burn unit. A SELAH volunteer visited her every day during the entire period. Not long after her release, another terrorist attack occurred. Many of the young soldiers were badly burned. Krakovich felt the need to reach out and help, to give back a part of what she had received from SELAH. Two years later, she described the process of transformation she experienced as a metamorphosis, relating, "After the caregiver seminar I went back to the same ward from which I had just come. The nurses pointed to me and said, 'Look how Anna is recovering.' I knew it was not only recovery. I had changed, like the trees we saw along the way."

The analogy of trees on a hilltop facing strong winds is an illustration of a useful metaphor from the caregiver seminars. This analogy was originally presented by Stephen Lepore and Tracey Revenson (Calhoun &Tedeschi, 1998), and has been elaborated by Stephan Joseph (2011). Some trees stand firm and unbending, while others may be snapped in half. Trees that bend to accommodate the wind may or may not recover and resume their original position. Other trees change shape and are permanently changed. "Lashed by the winds the tree will never be the same again, it grows around its injuries, and new leaves and branches sprout from the trunk of the tree where it had been severed. Scars, gnarls, and misshapen limbs give the tree its unique character. It is no less of a tree than it was, but it is different" (Joseph, 2011, p. 68).

Some trees may seem lifeless at first, yet still have the capacity for regeneration and nourishing new growth. Like the tree buffeted by the wind, people who grow following trauma might still remain emotionally affected, but their views on life, and their behaviors, will have changed in meaningful ways in light of their experiences.

A single mother, whose only daughter was killed in a suicide bombing, collected dry crumbling leaves and pieces of bark from the ground as she prepared a collage of scattered fragments loosely held together with a piece of rope. She placed a fig in the middle. She said, "Until yesterday, I felt that everything was dead within me, empty, like the dry bark. Everything was falling apart. Here you can see the shattered, scattered pieces. . . . This green fig is a sign of hope. Maybe."

Later she said that she was glad she had come, in spite of her initial reluctance, and told us how important it had been to her to reconnect to herself and her inner resources. She was proud of the work she prepared. "I am the eyes through which my daughter can look at the world," she said. "It is only through facing my own brokenness that I can help others reconnect to themselves and to life."

The language of metaphors crosses culture and language barriers. The use of metaphors facilitates the process of sharing experience by creating a communal language with which one can translate oneself to oneself and others. The group work provides caregivers with opportunities to tap into both individual and collective resources, and to identify the factors that can hinder their natural coping capacities, setting them up for burnout and compassion fatigue. Participants are encouraged to learn from one another and reflect on ways the practices shared in the seminars could expand their "toolboxes" by becoming fine-tuned, well-adapted, or simply more readily available to be applied when needed.

Figure 12.1 is a powerful picture and illustration of metaphors from nature.

Nature provides endless opportunities to learn about the cycles of change, life and death, as well as about processes of regeneration.

After the fire on the Carmel, in 2010, I gave a workshop in which participants had the opportunity to discuss burnout and regeneration. Resonating with the burned and cracked tree next to which the group was sitting, one of the volunteers, himself a bereaved parent whose son was killed in a terrorist

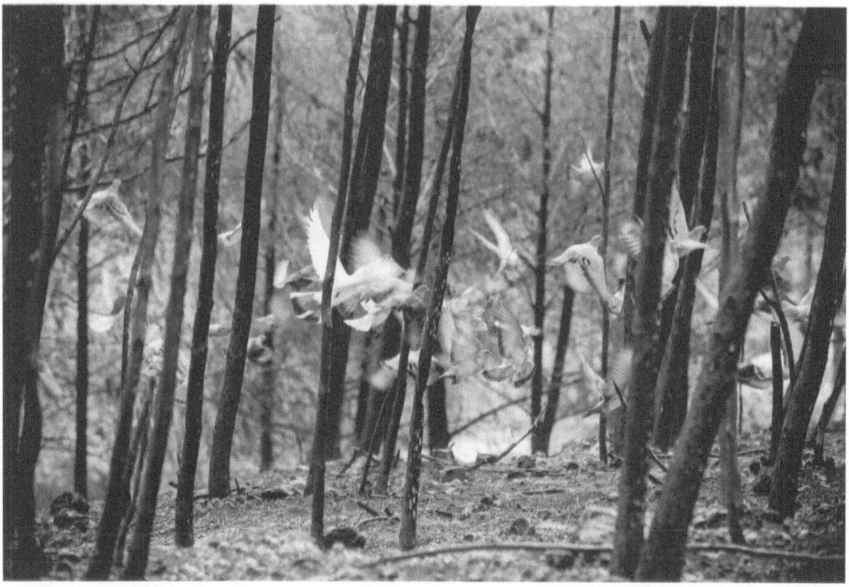

Figure 12.1. Rising from Ashes: Growth through adversity after the Carmel forest fire in December 2010. *Eleanor Pardess*

attack, talked about his experience of burnout—not only burning out, but also burning in (inside). Later on, he quoted Leonard Cohen, who he had met at a concert (the earnings from which went to the bereaved parents) when Cohen visited Israel in 2009. He resonated with the lines speaking about the deep crack within, and the struggle to connect. He felt a need to reach out to offer support the newly bereaved others ("We are all broken"). He added that he was not sure at first that he had anything to offer. "After my son was killed, I was surrounded by complete darkness. There was no meaning left, no reason to continue living. In the company of others, I learned to tie my tongue, to 'keep up a front.' I wanted to go on smiling, as I did before. However, I wasn't able to."

"All I could do was to just try and stretch my mouth into something that might pass as a smile. When I am alone, I feel that there is a black hole, an open vacuum in the place of my heart. Here in SELAH I don't have to hide my feelings, I can set my tongue free." The use of art enabled him to give sorrow shape.

He was worried that setting his tongue free would have devastating effect on other volunteers and that his own aching void would scare others, but discovered over time that "other bereaved parents understood what I was going through bur following "perfect offering, but a 'good enough.' I was surprised to discover the power of the group and actually found some comfort knowing others could understand what I was going through. We gain our strength from being together by sharing our stories and being part of a greater whole. They also seemed so strong on the outside like the burned tree on the way, but felt hollow and weak like I was." We had discussed good enough caregiving in the group.

He then sang the lines about how the light shines in the cracks of something that is broken. In other words, when something goes wrong, there is always a chance for transformation.

The group member could identify with the lines speaking about the deep crack within and the struggle to connect with and reach out to support the newly bereaved and help others. He felt that the training workshops, and the mutual support and understanding of others in the group, had helped him gather the strength to face his own wounded condition and darkness of suffering. Seeing the rays of light through the leaves of that olive tree reminded him of the cracks in his sense of self and home. Stepping out of his own personal isolated experience and connecting to nature and others in the group had a transformative effect for him, like seeing light through the cracks. He felt that he was part of a great human chain.

He then sang several lines of the song "Anthem" by Leonard Cohen.

The Experience of Being Uprooted

"We don't always have an opportunity to discover what goes on beneath the surface." With these words, the group stopped by a tree, the underground roots of which had been exposed and were intertwining by the side of the path. This workshop was held in a forest in the northern part of Israel. One of the participants, a single mother who had lost her only son in a suicide bombing, was particularly attracted to the severed root, which only she noticed. She bent over and gently stroked the root with emotion, remarking, "Just like my heart—broken in two." Later on, she drew a picture of the same tree with severed roots. She said, "I found myself identifying with the severed roots we saw on the way, split into two. On these roots there were green sprouts pushing their way out. Mine are now like those on the paper, only black. Yet, who knows? Maybe there will be growth in the future."

Another participant, who had noticed the way the roots of a tree grew around obstacles, commented, "People do not understand that we do not 'get over' a loss; rather, it becomes a part of us. It is with us all the time."

Keeping Roots Alive

Plants that have been uprooted, transplanted, and forced to adjust to new surroundings seem to have an inner knowledge of how to survive their relocation. At first, they invest all their energy in settling down and developing roots. During this stage they do not grow leaves or produce fruit, as that would be a waste of energy. The plant may seem to be "sick" or even "dead" on the outside, but the real story is what is going on under the surface. Underneath, roots are gradually developing and spreading out. It may be difficult to accept these periods in which there is no visible growth; however, it is important to know that this is not a waste of time but part of the process of rooting and grounding. Acclimatization takes time.

In a support group meeting for bereaved parents, a mother, whose 14-year-old daughter had been killed in a terrorist attack shortly after the family immigrated to Israel, told the group about the circumstances leading her to reach out and provide hope to others. Following her daughter's death, she tried to plant a cherry tree in Israel, using a sapling sent by her mother from the Ukraine—a tree like the one they had in their garden there. She reflected,

> It looked very sick and so sad here. We waited and waited. Not one leaf, not one flower. It was so dry. We thought it had already perished. One day my husband saw this tiny shoot pushing its way out. He is usually quite reserved, yet he was so excited, and even shouted in Hebrew (it was the first time he spoke a word of Hebrew at home), "Yesh, Yesh!"

The struggle of the tree resonated with the participants. "We also need care and nourishment, just like the plants," one of them commented. "And so much patience," said another. "I hate the word *savlanut* [patience in Hebrew], but I know deep inside that we have to be patient with all that is unresolved in ourselves."

The meaning of connecting to one's roots was elaborated on by group members. Some of them also commented on the different functions of roots that are essential for our nutrition and for firm anchorage. This discussion helped the caregivers maintain their own emotional equilibrium and weather the storms of life.

Trauma catapults people into the unknown. Anyone who has gone through trauma has asked themselves such searching questions as, Why me? What happened? What does it all mean? What do I do? Who am I? The answers do not always come easily, but when they do, they are potentially life-transforming. The combination of nature-based group experiences and the expressive arts opens new possibilities and creative ways for struggling with these questions and building bridges between the past, present, and future. Another key factor that fosters openness to emotion in promoting resilience and growth in these programs is the use of shared humor. The mindfulness practices foster emotional awareness and develop emotional tolerance.

Many caregivers find it practically impossible to attend to their own needs and well-being while caring for others. To provide validation and bear witness to pain, one has to be open to experiencing painful emotions; however, fears of emotional intensity may inhibit this ability. The experiential workshops can support the caregiver's tolerance of intense emotions by 1) making room for examining fears that emotions will be overwhelming and last indefinitely; 2) using mindful observation of emotions—that is, observing an emotion when it arises and not attempting to suppress or control it; and 3) providing caregivers with an opportunity to learn that their emotions not only "make sense," but also are a valuable source of information, and that stress can be an engine to growth (Joseph, 2011).

Long-term follow-ups and qualitative research have provided empiric support for the model. Caregivers report that following these workshops they do the following:

- Continue to reflect on these experiences and discover new strengths ("I feel that I've learned to ride the waves and discovered strengths I didn't know that existed").
- Respond to others in need with more awareness, rather than being on reactive "auto-pilot," and use that awareness to take whatever action will move them toward balance—as expressed in the comment, "This experi-

ence has enabled me to separate between my own feeling and that of others."

- Experience a sense of renewed commitment and compassion for themselves and others—as in the comment, "I used to be constantly worried that I am not doing enough, wondering if it is okay to feel so much pain and confusion. I feel more accepting toward myself now."

Resilience in the face of trauma exposure is not a static characteristic, but rather an individual's process of engagement with protective factors in the interaction between the self and the interpersonal environment. By enhancing intrapersonal and interpersonal self-awareness, caregivers can become more attentive to the presence of stress and their own personal capacity to find sources of nourishment and renewal.

The model developed in SELAH adds an additional dimension to current programs of cultivating growth and resilience by harnessing the power of metaphors from nature with the expressive arts and mindfulness practices. Moreover, this model converges with a whole-person approach by shifting away from conventional deficit-based models of trauma treatment and pathologizing discourses, and toward a comprehensive approach that promotes a view of our shared humanity, connectedness, resilience, and growth.

REFERENCES

Alkema, K., Linton, J. M., & Davies, R. (2008). A study of the relationship between self-care, compassion satisfaction, compassion fatigue, and burnout among hospice professionals. *Journal of Social Work in End-of-Life and Palliative Care*, *4*(2), 101–19.

Calhoun, L. G., & Tedeschi, R. G. (1998). Beyond recovery from trauma: Implications for clinical practice and research. *Journal of Social Issues*, *54*, 357–71.

Cocker, F., & Joss, N. (2016). Compassion fatigue among healthcare, emergency, and community service workers: A systematic review. *International Journal of Environmental Research and Public Health*, *13*, 618–35.

Craig, C. D., & Sprang, G. (2010). Compassion satisfaction, compassion fatigue, and burnout in a national sample of trauma treatment therapists. *Anxiety, Stress, and Coping*, *23*(3), 319–39.

Figley, C. R. (1995). *Compassion fatigue: Coping with secondary traumatic stress disorder in those who treat the traumatized*. New York: Brunner/Mazel.

Figley, C. R. (2002). *Treating compassion fatigue*. Psychosocial Stress Book Series. New York: Brunner/Routledge.

Joseph, S. (2011). *What doesn't kill us: The new psychology of posttraumatic growth*. New York: Basic Books.

Jung, C. G. (1961). *Memories, dreams, reflections*. New York: Random House.

Kopp, R. R. (1995). *Metaphor therapy: Using client-generated metaphors in psychotherapy*. New York: Brunner/Mazel.

Kornfield, J. (2008). *The wise heart: A guide to the universal teachings of Buddhist psychology*. New York: Bantam.

Kornfield, J. (1994). *Buddha's little instruction book*. London: Rider.

Lahad, M. (2000). Darkness over the abyss: Supervising crisis intervention teams following disaster. *Traumatology*, *6*(4), 273–93.

Lakoff, G., & Johnson, M. (2003). *Metaphors we live by*. London: University of Chicago Press.

Linley, P., & Joseph, S. (2007). Therapists' work and therapists' positive and negative well-being. *Journal of Social and Clinical Psychology, 26*, 385–40.

Lipsky, L. V. N. (2009). *Trauma stewardship: An everyday guide to caring for self while caring for others*. San Francisco, CA: Berrett-Koehler.

McCann, I. L., & Pearlman, L. A. (1990). Vicarious traumatization: A contextual model for understanding the effects of trauma on helpers. *Journal of Traumatic Stress, 3*, 131–49.

Neuschul, T., & Page, E. A. (2018). Creating shared worlds: Promoting mutual aid and community-building through expressive intervention. *Social Work with Groups, 41*(1/2), 21–33.

Pardess, E. (2005). Training and mobilizing volunteers in the aftermath of terrorist attacks. *Journal of Aggression, Maltreatment, and Trauma, 10*(1/2), 609–20.

Pardess, E., Mikulincer, M., Dekel, R., & Shaver, P. (2014). Dispositional attachment orientations, contextual variations in attachment security, and compassion fatigue among volunteers working with traumatized individuals. *Journal of Personality, 82*(5), 355–66.

Pearlman, L. A., & Caringi, J. (2009). Living and working self-reflectively to address vicarious trauma. In C. A. Courtois & J. D. Ford (eds.), *Treating complex traumatic stress disorders: An evidence-based guide* (pp. 202–24). New York: Guilford Press.

Remen, R. N. (1996). *Kitchen table wisdom: Stories that heal*. New York: Riverhead.

Rice, C. A. (2011). The psychotherapist as "wounded healer": A modern expression of an ancient tradition. In R. H. Klein, H. S. Bernard, & V. L. Schermer (eds.), *On becoming a psychotherapist: The personal and professional journey* (pp. 165–89). New York: Oxford University Press.

Rothschild, B. (2006). *Help for the helper: The psychophysiology of compassion fatigue and vicarious trauma*. New York: W. W. Norton.

Serlin, I. A. (2007). *Whole-person healthcare* (3 vols). Westport, CT: Praeger.

Serlin, I. A., & Cannon, J. T. (2004). A humanistic approach to the psychology of trauma. In D. Knafo (ed.), *Living with terror, working with trauma: A clinician's handbook* (pp. 313–30). Lanham, MD: Rowman & Littlefield.

Serlin, I. A., & Hansen, E. (2015). Stanley Krippner: Advocate for healing trauma. In J. A. Davis & D. B. Pitchford (eds.), *Stanley Krippner: A life of dreams, myths, and visions*. Colorado Springs, CO: University Professors Press.

Sodeke-Gregson, E. A., Holttum, S., & Billings, J. (2013). Compassion satisfaction, burnout, and secondary traumatic stress in UK therapists who work with adult trauma clients. *European Journal of Psychotraumatology, 4*(1), 1–10.

Tedeschi, R. G., & Calhoun, L. G. (1995). *Trauma and transformation: Growing in the aftermath of suffering*. Thousand Oaks, CA: Sage.

Vachon, M. L. S. (2015). Care of the caregiver: Professionals and family members. In J. M. Stillion & T. Attig (eds.), *Death, dying, and bereavement: Contemporary perspectives, institutions, and practices* (pp. 379–93). New York: Springer.

Wilkinson, M. (2017). Mind, brain, and body: Healing trauma: The way forward. *Journal of Analytical Psychology, 62*(4), 526–43.

Chapter Thirteen

Integrative Health Care of the Whole Person

Conclusion and Recommendations

Ilene Serlin, Stanley Krippner, and Kirwan Rockefeller

Having surveyed a group of original and powerful examples of interventions for people struggling with trauma, the editors chose to include working examples that exemplified different aspects of a whole-person approach. We did not attempt to be inclusive; an informed reader will easily identify a number of bases that were not covered. Nonetheless, each of the chapters in this book makes a unique contribution to the growing field of traumatology.

Rotter and Wertz's chapter describes a whole-person phenomenological research method that was used to understand and treat military trauma and the subsequent resilience. Their team discovered that the essential component of resilience is the soldier's ability to move flexibly between "soldier mode" and "civilian mode," and to recognize when such shifting serves important functions in daily life. Through a step-by-step exposition of their research method, they were also able to demonstrate the importance of methodological diversity in studying the lived experience of trauma.

As one of the first models of a working whole-person approach, the Meaningfulworld whole-person treatment plan is described by Kalayjian and Diakonova-Curtis. Developed by the Association of Trauma Outreach and Prevention (ATOP), its mission is to teach survivors how to make meaning from their traumatic experiences and forgive the perpetrators thereof. Both interventions are geared toward improving survivors' mental health, physical well-being, and spiritual development.

The creative arts therapies bring an aesthetic dimension to a whole-person approach. Thus, Kuriansky has employed art and play therapy with traumatized children in different parts of the world. Her chapter describes these workshops, which are whole person in nature by virtue of their integration of several psychosocial and psychoeducational interventions. Dance movement therapy (DMT) is another arts-based approach for working with trauma. Indeed, the chapter by Güney and Lundmark presents their whole-person work with asylum seekers by using DMT as a way of attending to the needs and circumstances of each group of survivors. Their program is holistic in that it provides care for the facilitators and includes a process of evaluation.

Engelman's chapter on animal-assisted intervention offers a whole-person approach that is biopsychospiritual in nature. Engelman's use of a dog or other animal as a cotherapist has been especially helpful for survivors whose condition is marked by withdrawal symptoms. Posttraumatic growth is built into the program from the beginning.

The Therapeutic Spiral Model (TSM), a drama-based intervention, is described by Israel as a clinically modified psychodramatic approach to working with people who have experienced trauma. TSM is anchored in psychodrama and experiential therapy, as well as clinical psychology and neuroscience. Spontaneity and creativity, which are at the core of TSM, are essential components of resilience.

Sword's chapter describes time-focused therapy, originally developed to assist military PTSD survivors but clearly applicable to other groups as well. It is a whole-person approach in that it is based on the existential dimension of time as a key element of the experience of trauma. Through a humanistic, collaborative endeavor, it promotes the healing of survivors through improving self-awareness, self-care, and social integration.

The potential power of using whole-person methods in communities was evident in several interventions. In their chapter, Recanati and associates discuss their NGO, NATAL, which serves as a multidisciplinary therapeutic home for trauma casualties related to the Israel–Arab conflict. The approach features a number of innovative whole-person modalities, for instance, the creative arts therapies, the use of nature, and a community-based hotline. In addition, NATAL provides safe spaces and ongoing support for family members and communities of those living with trauma. Since trauma in Israel is so pervasive, outreach into the community is essential.

Eshowsky's chapter illuminates how indigenous interventions for trauma include the interpersonal, community, historical, and spiritual contexts often missing from Western programs. Examining aspects of trauma understood by indigenous peoples as "soul loss," Eshowsky provides examples from contemporary restorative justice circles in South Africa and Cambodia. He also describes the application of the whole-person use of talking circles and rituals to work with trauma in local gang warfare and tribal conflicts in the United States.

In his chapter, Olweean articulates the Catastrophic Trauma Recovery (CTR) Model, which he has used to address survivors and their communities in the Middle East. The CTR Model may be considered a whole-person approach, as it requires survivors to acknowledge the totality of their traumatic experience, addresses both the quantitative (objective) and qualitative (subjective) dimensions of their trauma, emphasizes their cultural setting, and supports the capacity of their community to expand its own self-healing. The model, which includes a spiritual dimension, can be applied to individuals, groups, or communities.

The future of the whole-person approach is already appearing in some settings. For example, Pardess acknowledges the importance of secondary stresses associated with trauma, for example, compassion fatigue. Her whole-person program is geared toward preventing compassion fatigue and secondary trauma, while promoting caregiver satisfaction and regeneration. Her modalities are multidimensional, as the program uses mindfulness training, as well as excursions into nature that, upon reflection, are turned into metaphors. These metaphors serve as the basis for expressive art to help each participant find new growth.

We hope that an understanding and appreciation of the whole-person interventions we have collected for this book will lead to further development, evaluation, and research. Some mental health care providers may find the magnitude of the whole-person approach daunting; however, one does what one can, given that attending to the physical, attitudinal, emotional, social, and spiritual aspects of a traumatized person or group may seem like an overwhelming task. But simply being aware of the complexity of trauma may stimulate each affected person or group to seek alliances with other caregivers and local resources. While the challenge is obvious, the response is uncertain; nevertheless, the future of our fractured world clearly depends upon the sharing of compassion, empathy, and hope.

Index

About the Authors

CHAPTER 1: THE WHOLE-PERSON APPROACH TO INTEGRATED HEALTH CARE

Ilene Serlin, PhD, BC-DMT, is a licensed psychologist and registered dance/movement therapist in practice in San Francisco and Marin County. She is past president of the San Francisco Psychological Association, a fellow of the American Psychological Association, and past president of the Division of Humanistic Psychology. An Associated Distinguished Professor of Psychology at the California Institute of Integral Studies, Serlin taught at Saybrook University, Lesley University, UCLA, the New York Gestalt Institute, and the C. G. Jung Institute in Zurich. She is editor of *Whole Person Healthcare* (2007, 3 vols.); has written more than 100 chapters and articles on body, art, and psychotherapy; and is on the editorial boards of the *Journal of Humanistic Psychology*, *Arts & Health: An International Journal of Research, Policy and Practice*, the *Journal of Applied Arts and Health*, and the *Humanistic Psychologist*.

Stanley Krippner, PhD, is professor of psychology at Saybrook University and coauthor or coeditor of four books on war trauma. He is the recipient of the American Psychological Association Award for Distinguished Contributions to the Advancement of International Psychology and the Ashley Montagu Peace Award, presented to him by Common Bond Institute. Krippner is a fellow of several professional organizations, including the American Psychological Association, the Association for Psychological Science, the Society for the Scientific Study of Religion, the Society for the Scientific Study of Sexuality, and the American Society for Clinical Hypnosis. He is the recipient of the Lifetime Career Award of the Society for Humanistic Psychology and the International Association for the Study of Dreams. Krippner, a licensed addiction and substance abuse counselor, has given workshops on the treatment of PTSD nightmares in China, Russia, Mexico, Brazil, and the United States.

Kirwan Rockefeller, PhD, an adjunct faculty member at Saybrook University, teaches in both the College of Integrative Medicine and Health Sciences and the College of Social Sciences. He is coeditor of *Spirituality and Healthcare*, volume 2 of the three-volume *Whole Person Healthcare* (2007), and author of *Visualize Confidence: How to Use Guided Imagery to Overcome Self-Doubt* (2007).

CHAPTER 2: METHODOLOGICAL DIVERSITY IN THE STUDY OF TRAUMA TREATMENTS

Batya Rotter, PhD, EdM, is a clinical psychologist at Clalit Medical Services in Jerusalem, Israel. She received her doctorate from Fordham University in New York, and her master's degree in education at Harvard University in Cambridge, Massachusetts. Rotter has lived and practiced in the United States, India, Australia, and Israel, and specializes in the study of military resilience and trauma. She received a Fulbright Fellowship from the U.S. Department of State, a Boren Scholarship from the U.S. Department of Defense, and an Alumni Dissertation Grant from Fordham University to conduct her doctoral research in Israel with Israeli military servicemen using phenomenological methods. She currently lives in Israel with her husband and two children.

Frederick J. Wertz, PhD, professor of psychology at Fordham University, coedited *Advances in Qualitative Research in Psychology: Themes and Variations* (1987), edited *The Humanistic Movement: Recovering the Person in Psychology* (1994), and coauthored *Five Ways of Doing Qualitative Analysis: Phenomenological Psychology, Grounded Theory, Discourse Analysis, Narrative Research, and Intuitive Inquiry* (2011). He has served as editor of the *Journal of Phenomenological Psychology* and the *Bulletin of Theoretical and Philosophical Psychology*; guest editor of *The Humanistic Psychologist*; and president of the Society for Theoretical and Philosophical Psychology (APA Division 24), the Society for Humanistic Psychology (APA Division 32), and the Interdisciplinary Coalition of North American Phenomenologists. Wertz received the Rollo May Award from APA Division 32 and Fordham's Distinguished Teaching Award in Science and Outstanding Graduate Professor Award; he also chaired Fordham's Psychology, Communications, and Media Studies Department and Computer and Information Sciences Department. Wertz is the APA Council Representative of APA Division 24 and president of the Society for Qualitative Inquiry in Psychology.

CHAPTER 3: THE SEVEN-STEP INTEGRATIVE HEALING MODEL

Ani Kalayjian, EdD, DDL, RN-BC, BCETS, DSc (Hon), founder and president of the Association for Trauma Outreach and Prevention, Meaningfulworld, is a graduate of the Teachers College at Columbia University, with master's and doctoral degrees, as well as an honorary doctor of science degree from Long Island University, New York. A United Nations consultant since 1988, she has received an Alumni of the Year Award from the Teachers College at Columbia University, the ANA Human Rights Award, the APA Div. 52 Mentoring Award, and Humanitarian Awards from both the University of Missouri and the Pakistan Social Council. Kalayjian is author of an internationally acclaimed book titled *Disaster and Mass Trauma* (2009) and was chief editor of an international book titled *Forgiveness and Reconciliation: Psychological Pathways to Conflict Transformation and Peace Building* (2010). She was also chief editor of *Emotional Healing around the World: Rituals and Practices for Resilience and Meaning-Making* (2 vols., 2010), a meditation CD on ancestral healing and transforming generational trauma, and eight films on humanitarian outreach projects.

Daria Diakonova-Curtis, PhD, is a licensed clinical psychologist in the state of New York and a staff psychologist at CHE Behavioral Health Services in New York City. She completed an international postdoctoral fellowship at the Department of Psychology at St. Petersburg State University in St. Petersburg, Russia, where she worked on a NIH-funded international prevention study with women at risk for HIV. Diakonova-Curtis's research and clinical areas include gender issues affecting women's health and well-being, violence against women and sexual health, and trauma-informed therapy. She is the recipient of the Paul Werner Dissertation Award for her study of sexual assault perceptions among Russian adults, and APA's Division of International Psychology's Graduate Student Research Award. She completed her APA-accredited predoctoral internship in clinical psychology at the Institute for Multicultural Counseling and Education Services in Los Angeles, California, where she specialized in providing psychological services to immigrant populations from the former Soviet Union, Russia, Armenia, and the Middle East. Diakonova-Curtis is an active member of the Association for Trauma Outreach and Prevention, Meaningfulworld; representative of the APA's Division of International Psychology to APA's IPsyNet; and an elected member of the APA's Division of Psychotherapy Diversity Committee. She has served on the Editorial Student Review Board of

Psychology of Women Quarterly and made presentations at the United Nations and national and regional conferences.

CHAPTER 4: ART FOR HELPING CHILDREN HEAL IN CRISIS AND DISASTER

Judy Kuriansky, PhD, is an internationally known psychologist, humanitarian first responder, and award-winning journalist. At the United Nations, she is the main NGO representative of the International Association of Applied Psychology and the World Council for Psychotherapy, and chair of the Psychology Coalition of NGOs accredited there. She successfully advocated for including mental health and well-being in the United Nations Agenda 2030. An adjunct professor at the Teachers College of Columbia University, Kuriansky has engaged in many multicultural projects integrating resilience and arts in Africa, Haiti, Japan, and other countries. Her anthologies include *Living in an Environmentally Traumatized World: Healing Ourselves and Our Planet*, *Ecopsychology: The Intersection of Psychology and Environmental Protection*, and the recent *The Psychosocial Aspects of a Deadly Epidemic: What Ebola Has Taught Us*.

CHAPTER 5: DANCE MOVEMENT THERAPY FOR SOCIAL CHANVE

Seda S. Güney, RDMP, MA, is an ADMP, UK-registered dance movement psychotherapist, trained in London and based in Istanbul, where she established the first official dance movement therapy service at a local psychiatric hospital. She is a board member of the Arts Psychotherapies Association in Turkey. Having worked internationally with disadvantaged groups, Güney has developed and facilitated trainings and workshop programs for trauma rehabilitation with refugee children and adults. She is a lecturer on dance movement therapy at a conservatory and medical school in Istanbul. She works in the fields of social change, trauma rehabilitation, refugee relief, and education.

Danny S. Lundmark, MT-BC, BM, graduated from Berklee College of Music with a degree in music therapy. Having received his music therapist-board certified (MT-BC) credentials from the American Music Therapy Association, he is a member of the Turkish Music Therapy Association. Lundmark specializes in child growth and development, trauma rehabilitation, and adult psychiatric health. He works with children and refugee populations, lectures at a university music therapy training program, and leads music therapy sessions at a psychiatric hospital in Istanbul. He also conducts various workshops and training sessions both within and outside of Turkey.

CHAPTER 6: ANIMAL-ASSISTED INTERVENTIONS WITH THOSE WHO ARE TRAUMATIZED

Suzanne R. Engelman, PhD, BCB, FT, is a licensed health and clinical psychologist with a private practice in Laguna Niguel, CA. She specializes in working with patients and their families struggling with serious medical illnesses, death, dying, bereavement, and stress-related disorders. Engelman holds board certification, at the associate fellow level, in biofeedback (thermal, heart rate variability, respiratory, electrodermal, EMG); fellow certification in thanatology; certification as an animal-assisted therapist; and certification in the Treatment of Post-Combat Behavioral Health Program from Alliant University in San Diego, CA (2009). Engelman, who is on the medical staff at St. Joseph, Mission, and Laguna hospitals, is the author of numerous articles. She is also editor of *Life-Threatening Illness: Mind/Body Approaches*. In her free time, she likes to hike in the wilderness; meditate; and spend time with her family, friends, and two animal-assistance therapy dogs, Lizzy and CJ.

CHAPTER 7: THE THERAPEUTIC SPIRAL MODEL

Sylvia Israel, LMFT (mfc #31245), TEP, RDT/BCT, is a nationally certified psychodrama trainer, educator, practitioner (TEP), registered drama therapist/board certified trainer (RDT/BCT), and internationally certified trainer in trauma using the Therapeutic Spiral Model. She is a founding member of the Bay Area Moreno Institute and founder/past director of Bay Area Playback Theatre. Israel is on the faculty at the California Institute of Integral Studies and Kansas State University, and has presented at Spirit Rock Meditation Center. She is past president of the Northern California Chapter of the National Association of Drama Therapy and a fellow of the American Society of Group Psychotherapy and Psychodrama. A national and international trainer, Israel ensures that her work blends verbal therapy, psychodrama, and other expressive arts. She specializes in grief and loss, trauma, and childhood abuse recovery, and working with survivors of the Holocaust and their descendants. She maintains a private practice in Marin County and San Francisco, working with individuals, couples, and groups.

CHAPTER 8: TIME-FOCUSED PSYCHOTHERAPY

Rosemary Sword is a time perspective therapist in private practice in Maui, Hawaii. Trained in the Hawaiian psychology based on forgiveness, ho'oponopono ("to make right"), she has practiced this form of healing, which is part of her own heritage, for more than 25 years. Along with her husband, Richard Sword, she developed time perspective therapy (TPT) in 2008. Sword is coauthor of *The Time Cure* (with Philip Zimbardo and Richard Sword), published in English (2012), as well as Polish and German (2013), and Russian and Chinese (2014). She has also authored *The Time Cure Therapist Guidebook* (2014); *Time Perspective Theory; Review, Research, and Application, Essays Honoring Philip G. Zimbardo* (2015); and several psychological journal articles. She is author of popular blog columns for PsychologyToday.com and the European Union journal AppealPower.com, with more than 60 TPT-related articles published to date. Sword is founder/developer of Aetas: Mind Balancing Apps (Discoveraetas.com) and, along with Philip Zimbardo, is currently writing the sequel to *The Time Cure*.

CHAPTER 9: ISRAEL TRAUMA AND RESILIENCY CENTER—NATAL

Judith Yovel Recanati is a leading entrepreneur and social activist who devotes her time, resources, and life to strengthening and empowering Israeli society. Together with her late husband, Dr. Israel (Rolly) Yovel, she founded a family philanthropic foundation, the Gandyr Foundation, which aspires to assist in strengthening and empowering Israeli society by supporting and cultivating civil society organizations. In 1998, together with the late Dr. Yossi Hadar, Recanati founded NATAL, the Israel Trauma Center for Victims of Terror and War. She serves as the chairperson of NATAL, which focuses on the multidisciplinary treatment of Israeli victims of terror and war, emphasizing rehabilitation and improving quality of life. In addition, she is actively involved in forming a new model of Israeli philanthropy. A member of the Israeli branch of the Jewish Funders Network (JFN), Recanati chaired the March 2015 JFN conference; she is also a board member at Sheatufim. Holding degrees in archeology and photography, she studied art therapy at Lesley College and psychotherapy at Bar Ilan University.

CHAPTER 10: INDIGENOUS HEALING PSYCHOTHERAPY AND RESTORATIVE CIRCLES

Myron Eshowsky, MS, counseling psychology, is a counselor, shamanic healer, mediator, and educator. He is codirector of the Social Health Care

Program for Syrian Refugees, which provides direct services and training in trauma treatment for refugees in the Middle East. He has consulted throughout the United States and internationally, addressing the trauma healing needs in gangs, youth at risk, prisons, and communities traumatized by violence, notably historical trauma, and child soldiers in Africa.

CHAPTER 11: WHOLE-PERSON APPROACHES IN INDIVIDUAL AND COMMUNAL HEALING OF TRAUMA

Steve S. Olweean, MA, is founding director of the Common Bond Institute (CBI); founding president of the International Humanistic Psychology Association; past president of the Association for Humanistic Psychology (AHP); the recipient of various awards, notably the 2011 Charlotte and Karl Bühler Award from the APA Div. 32, for outstanding and lasting contributions to humanistic psychology internationally; and a therapist with a degree in clinical psychology from Western Michigan University in Kalamazoo, Michigan. For 15 years he led the AHP Soviet–American Professional Exchange. Olweean has more than 40 years of experience in community-based mental health treatment of high-risk populations. Near the end of the Balkan Wars, he developed the integrated Catastrophic Trauma Recovery (CTR) model for treating large traumatized populations. The CTR model is the basis for CBI's whole-person Social Health Care training and treatment program, which equips local Middle Eastern students, NGO staff, and refugees with trauma-informed skills to assist impacted populations, promote a resilient self-help community identity, and develop local human service and academic systems. Olweean has been an activist in the human rights and peace movements since his university student years, a commitment and experience that continue to inform his work today.

CHAPTER 12: PROMOTING CAREGIVER SATISFACTION AND REGENERATION

Eleanor Pardess, MA, PhD, is a clinical psychologist and trauma specialist working in Tel-Aviv, Israel. She has created Moving Encounters, which is a multimodal model of facilitating posttraumatic growth. She uses this model at SELAH, the Israel Crisis Management Center, and in training and mobilizing volunteers for emergencies. Pardess also teaches this model about trauma and the lifecycle at the School of Social Work at Tel Aviv University and at the Interdisciplinary Center in Herzliya. Her research also focuses on compassion fatigue and regeneration.

CHAPTER 13: INTEGRATIVE CARE OF THE WHOLE PERSON: CONCLUSION AND RECOMMENDATIONS

See biographies of the editors for chapter 1.

www.ingramcontent.com/pod-product-compliance
Ingram Content Group UK Ltd.
Pitfield, Milton Keynes, MK11 3LW, UK
UKHW012038150926
475560UK00001B/76

9 781538 121375